The Newly Qualified Paramedic's Handbook

This book is dedicated to the first patient I treated as a qualified paramedic, who nearly died. They didn't, not because of me but because of the entire team involved in their treatment – from the bystander who found them and called for help promptly, the 999 emergency medical advisor who took the call and gave clear pre-arrival instructions, the technician I was working with who knew my job better than I did, the triage nurse who cleared a resus bed based on little more than the non-verbal clues in my radio priority message, to the extensive team of hospital staff who provided the definitive care that I had just about started. It takes a system to save a life, and working safely and effectively within that system is the greatest skill a person can learn.

The Newly Qualified Paramedic's Handbook

Transitioning to Independent Practice

Danny Dixon

CLASS
Professional

Printing history

This edition first published in 2026.

The authors and publisher welcome feedback from the users of this book.

Please contact the publisher:

Class Professional Publishing,
The Exchange, Express Park, Bristol Road, Bridgwater TA6 4RR
Telephone: 01278 472 800
Email: info@class.co.uk
Website: www.classprofessional.co.uk

Class Professional Publishing is an imprint of Class Publishing Ltd

A CIP catalogue record for this book is available from the British Library

Paperback ISBN: 9781801611329
ePub ISBN: 9781801611336
ePDF ISBN: 9781801611343

Cover design by Nicky Borowiec
Designed and typeset by S4Carlisle Publishing Services

Refer to local recycling guidance on disposal of this book.

Product safety information can be found at https://www.classprofessional.co.uk/terms-of-use/gpsr-statement/

Contents

Acknowledgements

This book would not exist without the practical and emotional support of a huge number of people. Firstly, to the team at Class Professional Publishing, and in particular the editor of this book Katherine Totterdell, thank you for taking a chance on me and guiding me through the process as a novice author.

Secondly, to my colleagues and friends who have supported me through my clinical and educational career. Thank you for the support, encouragement and regular reality checks to get me to this stage – I am grateful to all of you.

Lastly, to my family. Thank you to my wife, Hannah, who has been a constant presence, one of encouragement, reassurance and support – I love you. And to my children, Joshua and Tabitha, who have taught me nothing about being a paramedic but everything about being a better person. This book, and everything, is for you.

About the Author

Danny Dixon is a passionate and experienced paramedic, with a background in education and staff development and an interest in using his skills and experience to further the careers of others. He loves to learn, and loves to share that learning with others – with a strong focus on restorative culture and continuous improvement.

He is currently working as Head of Community Resilience at South East Coast Ambulance Service. He has previously worked as Senior Education Manager at the same Trust, as well as undertaking paramedic lecturer roles at various universities across the South East. He remains the Trust's subject matter expert for supporting newly qualified paramedics and the preceptorship programme.

Danny trained as a paramedic at St George's, University of London in Tooting, and undertook his Postgraduate Certificate in Academic Practice at Canterbury Christ Church University. He lives in Surrey with his wife, Hannah, two children and their cat.

Abbreviations

ACP – advanced clinical practitioner

AHP – allied health profession(al)

CPD – continuing professional development

CFR – community first responder

CRM – crew resource management

CQC – Care Quality Commission

EBP – evidence-based practice

GP – general practitioner (primary care doctor)

HCP – healthcare professional

HCPC – Health and Care Professions Council

JESIP – Joint Emergency Services Interoperability Programme

JRCALC – Joint Royal Colleges Ambulance Liaison Committee

NHS – National Health Service

NQP – newly qualified paramedic

PAD – practice assessment document

PAP – private ambulance provider

PEd – practice educator

PSRB – professional, statutory and regulatory bodies

SET – Standards of Education and Training

SOP – scope of practice

Introduction

Completing your paramedic course and starting work in your chosen profession as a Newly Qualified Paramedic (NQP) is exciting – you finally get to put into practice all the skills and techniques you have spent a significant amount of time developing. It can also be terrifying – suddenly as a new registrant you become accountable for the decisions you make, and responsible for the physical and emotional wellbeing of both patients and colleagues. This book aims to guide you through the first couple of years of your clinical practice, as you make the transition from student, to newly qualified, and ultimately to experienced paramedic.

The rapid expansion of the paramedic profession has led to greater diversity in the potential working environment for NQPs than ever before. This, coupled with efficiency savings within the National Health Service affecting recruitment, means the ambulance service is no longer viewed as the default choice for many graduating student paramedics. For some this can be a cause of anxiety, but it can also be an opportunity to explore other areas where paramedicine may be a less established, but equally rewarding area of healthcare. What hasn't changed is the importance of encouragement, guidance and support during the formative years of your career, and whether you start your career in an ambulance service alongside other NQPs, or choose to work in a less familiar clinical setting, this book aims to provide you with the confidence, information and resilience to excel. From your first shift to your first setback, this book includes practical tips on bridging the gap between theory and practice and consolidating the wealth of knowledge you have gained as a student into professional and proactive patient care.

Throughout the book are reflective activities, designed to support you to deepen your understanding of the key topics discussed, and build on your existing knowledge. For those completing the national Consolidation of Learning Programme for NQPs, these activities align with the learning outcomes of that programme. For those developing independently or undertaking other programmes, they will provide a varied range of continuing professional development to support the requirements of employers and the Health and Care Professions Council (HCPC).

Finally, the book contains a range of insights and advice from students, newly qualified and experienced paramedics to allow you to benefit from their experiences and to provide additional context. These can also be used to provoke your own individual reflections as you undertake the journey from novice to expert. Although your own path from student to experienced paramedic will be unique, it is a journey which has been undertaken by many others, all of whom can help support you with your development.

Chapter 1
Choosing a Post as a Newly Qualified Paramedic

The College of Paramedics (2024a) defines a paramedic at the point of registration as:

> 'an independent, graduate-level, generalist clinician commencing a journey of lifelong learning. Approaching their patients holistically, they draw on a range of systems-based assessments, diagnostic tools, and interventional skills; and are able to manage an undifferentiated, diverse, and complex case-load of patients, including the critically ill and injured, doing so in environments over which they have limited control. They advocate for their patients, stratifying risk and navigating changeable health and care systems to implement appropriate person-centred management plans autonomously, and as part of a multidisciplinary team. They support and supervise colleagues, as well as seek advice and support when needed. They exhibit professional values, attributes, skills and knowledge across the four domains of practice that are underpinned by ethical reasoning, research and evidence.'

That's a lot to unpack in one paragraph, but this description could be summarised as a *Johannes factotum* or a jack-of-all-trades — a generalist clinician who is comfortable working across diverse environments, at various stages in the patient journey and in different areas of the healthcare system. With such versatility, it is perhaps unsurprising that the National Health Service (NHS) Long Term Workforce Plan (2023) identifies a need to increase the paramedic workforce at both graduate and advanced levels, as well as increasing opportunities for paramedics to learn and work across hospital, community and primary care settings. In practice, this means that employment opportunities for newly qualified paramedics (NQPs) are more diverse than ever, although the number of posts will inevitably vary with the political climate and funding availability.

Employment Options for Newly Qualified Paramedics

Despite the high demand for paramedics across both public and private healthcare, the majority of NQPs still prefer to start their careers within an ambulance service, and for good reason – there are few other working environments which can offer the same range of patient presentations and degree of autonomous practice as an ambulance service. The ambulance environment likely encapsulates much of what first attracted you to the paramedic role, and over three-quarters of paramedics nationally will continue to work in an ambulance setting (HCPC, 2021).

Working in an ambulance service offers you the opportunity to consolidate the knowledge and skills you have gained during your paramedic course. As the biggest employers of paramedics, ambulance services also provide valuable opportunities to continue learning while working alongside other more experienced colleagues. This is embodied in a national consolidation of learning programme which all NHS ambulance services are committed to delivering. While terminology and application may vary, the underlying principles remain consistent. Preceptorship is discussed further in Chapter 2, but the benefits of the support offered should not be overlooked.

An NHS ambulance service may not be the favoured option for all NQPs, and personal circumstances, job availability or career ambitions may encourage you to consider other working environments, some of which are discussed below.

Private Ambulance Providers (PAP)

There are a vast number of PAPs providing services across the country, ranging from event medical cover and patient transport services to sub-contracted emergency ambulance responses for the NHS.

Considerations

Working for a PAP may provide more flexibility, greater variety of work opportunities, and chances to travel across different locations, while per hour pay can be higher than in the NHS. However, employment benefits (sickness protection, pension) may not be as favourable and support for employees varies. There have also been several high-profile closures which have left staff without employment (Express and Star, 2023; Kent Online, 2024).

Tip

Always be clear on the terms and conditions of employment prior to accepting a role and compare these to alternative employers – particularly whether they offer a preceptorship programme which aligns to NHS trusts.

Alternatives

- Event medical services
- Film and television sets.

Primary Care

General practitioner (GP) surgeries are increasingly enthusiastic about employing NQPs, either as clinicians in their own right or as part of a development pathway towards advanced clinical practitioner (ACP). You may be asked to undertake clinics, home visits, patient reviews or telephone consultations.

Considerations

Primary care often offers a clear development pathway to advanced practice, although this does vary by employer and is worth exploring at application. Clinical supervision is generally well established with the opportunity to learn from a multidisciplinary team, but if your experience of primary care is limited you may find that your expectations don't match reality, particularly in terms of the acuity of the workload and time pressures for patient consultations.

Tip

Discuss with the practice in advance what the scope of practice will be and the support available for the role.

Prison Service

The prison environment offers a unique opportunity to undertake a mixture of primary and acute care within a secure environment. You may also experience the balance of being the sole paramedic while working within a multidisciplinary team, great for support and learning opportunities. Although prisons rarely seek NQP appointments, there are opportunities advertised which don't specify a requirement for experience.

Considerations

A unique environment offering a balance of autonomy and support, with the likelihood of clinical exposure to a range of acute and emergency patient presentations. However, you may risk isolation as a clinical lead.

Tip

Working in a prison setting requires confidence and the ability to work independently. A compassionate approach and strong communication skills are essential.

Alternatives

- Forensic paramedic within a custody suite.

Remote/Expedition Medicine

There are a range of hazardous environments that people travel to for the purposes of leisure, business or security, many of which require a healthcare professional (HCP) to travel alongside the team or remain at a nearby location. Increasingly, paramedics are recruited to these posts, although the exact requirements will depend on the location and specific risks.

Considerations

Opportunities are often varied, offering unique travel experiences. The nature of healthcare provided can also vary considerably (this can be a benefit or a risk), with limited or no support for decision making or secondary care. There may be a requirement or opportunity for specialist qualifications, and employment may be seasonal.

Tip

Consider the location first and the clinical role second – if the environment is not appealing, it is unlikely to be enhanced by working as an NQP.

Alternatives

- Remote location healthcare sites
- Gas and oil rigs
- Personal protection teams
- Medical repatriation.

Lecturing

As the profession becomes increasingly academic, universities are employing NQPs directly into faculty positions, sometimes as part of a Master's or doctoral pathway.

Considerations

If you are interested in education or research, this is an excellent way to influence the future of the profession, but without the simultaneous opportunity to practise clinically, it may be harder to traverse the 'theory–practice' divide which can reduce academic credibility.

Tip

Consider gaining experience in a clinical setting alongside teaching activity, to ensure sufficient experience to answer the tricky 'what if' questions.

Alternatives

- Teaching positions in other settings (such as first aid)
- Health provider in schools
- Ambulance service teaching posts.

Overseas Ambulance Services

For those who are seeking new challenges or experiences outside of the UK, applying for an ambulance service overseas may be appealing. Although vacancies and relocation packages vary, many services recognise the benefit of recruiting clinicians from a diverse range of backgrounds.

Considerations

Although Emergency Medical Services (EMS) can be found throughout the world, there are significant variations in the operating model each follows, often depending on the geographical and socio-economic circumstances of the country in which they are based, and whether there is a national healthcare system in place (either publicly or privately funded). Take time to carefully research both the EMS provision and the wider healthcare system, as well as lifestyle and logistical considerations such as cost of living, visa or work permit requirements, professional registration expectations, language barriers, and availability of a support network.

Tip

Consider enlisting the support of a professional relocation company to help with the administration of relocating overseas for work. To support with the decision, online forums offer the opportunity to learn from the experiences of others who have made similar moves.

Alternatives

There are many possible countries to choose from, but areas such as Canada, Australia, New Zealand and the United Arab Emirates have all recruited paramedics from the UK previously.

Others

There are plenty of other settings now employing NQPs, each with unique benefits and risks. These include:

- Medical teams on cruise ships
- Armed forces

- Hospital wards and emergency departments
- Healthcare research
- Residential care homes and hospices
- Self-employment.

Often it is possible to undertake these roles on a part-time or 'bank' basis alongside a full-time role elsewhere, but if doing so you must remain aware of employer policies on secondary employment and ensure adequate insurance cover.

Tip

The College of Paramedics Interactive Career Framework (cop-icf.co.uk) showcases the variety of paramedic roles available and may act as a source of inspiration.

Returning to the NHS Ambulance Service

A common concern amongst NQPs who do consider working elsewhere, either immediately following graduation or during their first two years, is whether they will be able to return to the ambulance service in the future, and, if so, at which grade. The simple answer is that while the details will depend on individual circumstances, working in another environment will never be a barrier to being appointed to an NHS ambulance service, and the added experience gained will probably be looked upon favourably at application. Whether a Trust offers you a post as an NQP (band 5) or an experienced (band 6) paramedic will depend on the amount of and relevance of the experience you have gained in other roles, and whether you can evidence completion of a preceptorship programme. Both these considerations will be linked to the requirements of the role's job description. It is worth considering that even where there is a requirement to re-enter the NHS in a band 5 NQP role, all ambulance services now follow a national 'fast track' process to allow previous experience to be considered and having a varied breadth of experience may be beneficial for your future career progression opportunities.

Applying For, and Being Offered, a Job

One of the first barriers to overcome before working as an NQP is landing a job in the role, which for some can be a nerve-racking or stressful process in its own right. Although many NQPs are offered the opportunity to work in the ambulance Trust where they have undertaken student practice placements, this usually still involves a recruitment process. Alternatively, you may explore work opportunities elsewhere, either due to geographical considerations (for example, to return to the familial home), the particular appeal of a specific ambulance Trust, or the desire to work in a different environment altogether.

Regardless of the employer, how you approach the assessment process can set the tone for your future career, and while the availability of paramedic posts remains variable depending on the prevailing financial and political climate, applying for desirable roles or areas is likely to remain a competitive process.

Preparing an Application

Before applying for any role, it is important to ensure you meet the necessary criteria. Most job descriptions include a person specification section, which will identify both the 'essential' and 'desirable' requirements for the role. Outside of the ambulance service, it is less likely that jobs will differentiate suitability for the NQP, but they may require evidence of post-registration experience in the clinical setting or as a clinical lead, which can exclude NQPs. While it may seem tempting to embellish accomplishments or simply ignore unmet aspects of the essential criteria, this is unprofessional and often leads to frustration for both you and the recruiting organisation. Where there is any doubt about suitability, it is sensible to contact the recruiting organisation first (most job adverts will have relevant contact details). This allows for an open, two-way discussion about the expectations of the potential employer and can either save time or reinforce suitability. It also demonstrates a professional and honest work ethic, which will always be appreciated.

Once eligibility has been determined, the next stage is to prepare your application. Again, organisations vary in terms of how they receive applications, which may be through a standardised application form, submission of a resumé or curriculum vitae (CV), or through an online recruitment management system. Whichever method is used, it is important you follow instructions and complete forms carefully. Online systems (particularly when undertaking bulk recruitment) will often specifically request that you do not submit a CV, and doing so may result in your application being rejected. Some systems will utilise screening questions to ensure applicants are suitable. Where your answer may not meet the eligibility criteria (for example, when applying for a job while still a student and therefore not yet registered with the HCPC), there may be an option for 'pending', but if not then answer honestly. If this causes your application to be rejected, contact the recruiting organisation directly to discuss.

Finally, it is common to be asked to provide 'supporting information' or a 'personal statement'. This is your opportunity to demonstrate why you are the best person for the role beyond the basics of meeting the essential person specification, and should therefore be evidence based, using your experiences to demonstrate how you meet the competencies.

ACTIVITY

Write a brief supporting statement based on your current qualifications and experience. Leave it for a few weeks, then read it again from the perspective of an employer. Would you hire yourself? What changes can you make to enhance your profile? Once you have completed this exercise you can save the information to use or adapt for CPD, resumés or job applications.

ADVICE

'When writing a job application, print a copy of the person specification and physically tick off the list when each element is evidenced — that way none get missed.'

Interview and Assessments

Once an application has been shortlisted, you will usually be invited to an interview or other assessment process (see Table 1.1 for examples). Interviews may be a mixture of competency or values based – competency-based interviews generally expect you to share an experience where you have demonstrated the element being assessed ('tell me about a time that...') whereas values-based questions are more likely to ask about a hypothetical situation ('what would you do if...'). It is common for people to become nervous during interviews, which can cause either a difficulty with forming cohesive sentences or conversely a tendency towards verbosity which can be repetitive or irrelevant to the question. Both these risks can be mitigated by using a simple structure to formulate interview responses. One such structure is the STAR technique (Lark, 2023):

- **S**ituation: what is the background or context of the event – briefly!
- **T**ask: what was your specific goal?
- **A**ction: what steps did *you* (not others) take to reach this goal?
- **R**esults: what was the outcome – keep it positive and take credit for your work.

This can be supplemented by adding a further T, to make START:

- **T**akeaways: what you have learned from the experience.

An alternative structure is useful specifically when discussing issues or difficulties that you have faced, and can be remembered as 3 Rs:

- **R**ecognise: how did you identify and isolate the issue?
- **R**ectify: what did *you* (not others) do to resolve this issue?
- **R**esults: what was the impact of your actions on the issue, and your future learning?

Table 1.1 – Types of assessment.

Assessment	Preparation for success
Driving assessment	Ask what type of vehicle will be used for assessment (size, weight, gearbox). Consider hiring a similar vehicle to practise. Use online or app-based highway code tests. Seek support from driving instructor.
Clinical simulation	Have confidence in experience gained. Undertake peer practice sessions. Review national clinical practice guidelines – employers will not expect familiarisation with internal guidelines.
Physical fitness assessment	Ask what the expected standard is. Simple but consistent exercise is often sufficient – be prepared to maintain this; fitness levels will not change overnight. Cardiovascular exercise (anything which increases heart rate) is often most beneficial. Consult a GP regarding any specific health concerns. Speak to advisors at local gyms.
Psychometric tests	Psychometric testing is increasingly popular to provide an unbiased and objective overview of candidate aptitude, but there is limited preparation which is beneficial. The best results are obtained by remaining calm and composed while completing the test, which can be augmented by familiarity with the testing method. To support this, it is possible to find a range of sample tests online.

One of the most common worries about interviews is fear of the unknown – not knowing what interview questions you will be asked. While this is an understandable concern, no matter how the question is phrased the interviewer will be trying to gain information about you linked to a particular theme, and nobody knows more about you than you do!

✎ ACTIVITY

With a friend or peer, create a mind map of the subjects or themes which are most likely to appear in a paramedic interview, and then in turn ask each other possible interview questions. Constructively critique the responses.

Reasonable Adjustments

When applying for a new role, the same moral and legal imperatives to ensure a fair process and prevent discrimination exist as for someone already in employment (Equality Act 2010). While there is no requirement to inform a potential employer about any disabilities, it may be that you require reasonable adjustments to ensure fairness during the recruitment process. This may be particularly relevant if you are neurodiverse, but applies to all types of disability and other protected characteristics. Requests for reasonable adjustments should be discussed directly with the recruiting organisation, clearly explaining the reason why the adjustment is needed and what is most likely to assist.

💬 ADVICE

'Discuss reasonable adjustments early – it can reduce some of the stress associated with attending an interview, and in the unlikely event that an organisation is unsupportive, it is better to find out before committing to work there.'

Receive, Review and Respond

Following a successful interview or assessment, the next stage is to receive a job offer. This may be verbal initially but should be followed up in writing. Once received, take the time to review the offer carefully. It may be either a conditional offer (where progressing to employment is dependent on certain conditions being met) or unconditional. Either way, at this stage once you accept the offer it is legally binding and cannot be withdrawn except under specific circumstances. It is prudent to check the offer is as expected, particularly regarding details such as salary, base location, working hours and benefits. If any details are unclear, clarify before accepting the offer – most employers appreciate applicants who take a professional approach to understanding the terms of employment.

Once the terms are agreed, respond in writing to formally accept and start completing any pre-employment administration, checks or paperwork required.

Flexible Working

Requests for flexible working are increasingly common as the employment landscape becomes more family friendly. The NHS England (2024) offers the right for NHS employees to request flexible working from their first day of employment. This could include part-time working, annualised hours, fixed shifts or other adjustments. It is important to note, however, that organisations are only required to consider requests and not obliged to accept them, particularly where they are not practicable to implement, although where requests are declined a reasonable explanation should be provided. Ultimately, if you require specific flexible working agreements, it is important these are discussed and formally agreed prior to accepting a job offer.

> 💬 **ADVICE**
>
> 'Always ensure any specific agreements with a new employer are confirmed in writing – if discussed by telephone, ask for this to be followed up by email.'

> ✏️ **ACTIVITY**
>
> Make a list of all the considerations, attributes, employment terms and working conditions which would make up your ideal post as an NQP. Next, use the MoSCoW prioritisation method (Clegg and Barker, 1994) to sort these into four categories: **M**ust have, **S**hould have, **C**ould have and **W**on't have. This can help determine where to work and encourage rational compromise.

Choosing Where to Work

When considering options, it is important to choose a job which allows you to thrive rather than simply survive. Concerns around longevity of service for paramedics are well documented. High workload, emotional stress, poor mental health and the challenges of performing the role to the aspired high standard all contribute to high sickness levels and staff turnover, while the availability of greater clinical challenges offered elsewhere in the NHS are often alluring (Hayes, 2022). Crucially, however, it may be the experiences within an ambulance service which are perceived as negative which best prepare paramedics to excel in other clinical settings – with seemingly 'mundane' low-acuity presentations developing your patient assessment, remote working promoting autonomy and independent decision making, and austere environments fostering confidence and clinical courage (Mallinson, 2020). As an NQP, there is both an enthusiasm and need to develop these skills, since 'no undergraduate curriculum could reasonably hope to capture such range of clinical opportunity available for the profession in the 21st century' (Eaton, 2023).

It is therefore wise that when looking for employment, you first seek to understand the support available to you within your prospective workplace, including who will be providing that support. Key considerations should include the following:

- *Number of NQPs recruited each year*: aside from 'safety in numbers', this provides an indication of how experienced the employer is in supporting paramedics in general, and those that who are newly qualified specifically.

- *Who will be your clinical supervisor*: although there are benefits to working as part of a multi-disciplinary team, this should be balanced against the reassurance of having a direct clinical supervisor with the same clinical role and background.

- *How long the organisation has been recruiting paramedics*: are paramedics an established part of the workforce or a new development which is not yet fully embedded? It can be hard to focus on personal development as a new practitioner if there is a simultaneous need to develop the representation of the profession.

- *Is there an established preceptorship programme*: what specific support is available for you, considering whether this is focused specifically on paramedics or for allied health professionals (AHP), and how transferable it is likely to be between organisations.

It is not unreasonable to ask about these details either at application or interview stage, and your decision to take on a new post should be based on the relative merits of all these factors.

Chapter 2
What is Preceptorship?

Compared to the complexity of clinical practice, plants may be considered simple, uncomplicated and plain, but the process of photosynthesis which allows plants (and by extension, all other life) to flourish is deceptively intricate. Rather than soil, sunlight is the key nutrient without which no plant can survive. The key takeaway is that no plant can flourish purely from a solid grounding, the environment is also fundamental to growth.

The same can be said of NQPs. At the point of registration, the sense of achievement is justifiably significant, but this is merely the roots of future development. It is your application of this learning, and by extension the working environment in which your consolidation takes place, which has the greatest impact on progress. It follows that proactive and positive support during this period is essential. Preceptorship is the mechanism through which this support can, and should, be provided.

Defining Preceptorship

Preceptorship is a structured mentorship period for NQPs. In practice, this means that a new graduate is paired with an experienced practitioner (a preceptor) who provides one-on-one guidance, feedback and role modelling on the job. The concept of a 'preceptor' originates from the 15th century, meaning a teacher who focuses on sharing 'precepts' (principles governing conduct, actions or procedures), as distinct from traditional teaching programmes which concentrate on knowledge and skills acquisition. This hands-on support helps bridge the gap between classroom learning and real patient care. Regulators and the NHS now expect that new clinicians receive this support when they start work. In 2023 NHS England launched the Allied Health

Professions Preceptorship Standards and Framework with the aim of 'empowering new beginnings and building confidence for AHPs transitioning into new roles or workplaces' (NHS England, 2023a).

> **✏️ ACTIVITY**
>
> Before starting a preceptorship programme, consider how you would most like to develop, both personally and professionally. Instead of focusing on specific actions (a 'to do' list), write yourself a 'to be' list – where would you like to be at the end of your preceptorship? Save this in your portfolio and review in two years to see what you have achieved.

From Novice to Expert

The Department of Health (2008) defines preceptorship as 'a foundation period for practitioners at the start of their career to help them begin the journey from novice to expert, enabling them to apply the professionalism, knowledge, skills and competencies acquired as students into their area of practice, and laying a solid foundation for life-long learning'. That journey from novice to expert is described by Benner (1984) as the progression of any healthcare practitioner as they develop competence within a specific field (Table 2.1).

Dr Patricia Benner based her work on the Dreyfus Model of Skills Acquisition and applied this initially to the field of nursing. She recognised that gaining expertise takes time – as important as education is, applying learning in a clinical setting is what allows practitioners to develop. Although critics would argue that Benner's model is too linear, the stages are not intended to be prescriptive but instead you will probably move between different stages at different times depending on the area of practice you are developing. A simple example of this can be considered by comparing clinical practice with leadership – both are important, but you are likely to progress in your clinical practice more rapidly due to more frequent opportunities for exposure, which is required to improve competency.

Table 2.1 – Benner's (1984) stages of proficiency.

Stage	Definition	Application
Novice	Beginner with no experience. Rules-based approach to actions and decision. Direct supervision required.	Undergraduate paramedic student. Works well under instruction to develop technical skills.
Advanced beginner	Sufficient clinical practice experience to recognise patterns. Begins to make decisions by applying these patterns to guidelines.	NQP at point of registration. Relies heavily on clinical practice guidelines but generally recognises appropriate guideline.
Competent	Actions are seen in terms of longer-term goals. Applies abstract and analytical principles to plan effectively and efficiently.	NQP with 1–2 years' experience. Starts to anticipate and plan for patient needs during, rather than following, patient assessment.
Proficient	Uses incomplete information to see whole situation. Applies maxims to decision making.	Experienced paramedic. Effectively mentors and supports others.
Expert	Intuitive and holistic understanding and decision making, beyond rules, maxims or guidelines.	Highly experienced or specialist paramedic. Rapidly and safely interprets situations and sees beyond existing standards.

It is unlikely that you will become an expert, or even fully proficient, during your preceptorship; however, you will probably develop areas of interest or microspecialties where you may demonstrate expertise. It is important to note that preceptees are recognised as safe but inexperienced practitioners, undertaking the first step in career-long development rather than addressing any deficit in training or ability. Therefore, preceptorship should be seen as a model of enhancement providing a supportive scope of practice as a safeguard while proficiency develops, rather than a restrictive environment which withholds autonomy.

Benefits of Preceptorship

The longer-term benefits of completing preceptorship apply to both the NQP and the employing organisation. NHS Ambulance Service paramedics are somewhat unique amongst AHPs, insofar as the conclusion of preceptorship heralds an automatic promotion into the experienced paramedic role; in addition to a pay rise, this also results in a higher level of responsibility, particularly supervisory responsibility and autonomous decision making. Preceptorship should prepare you for this, ensuring you are confident and competent to take on the new aspects of your role independently, through hands-on experience and the development of critical thinking. It also ensures you are professionally socialised into the culture of your organisation, that you fully understand the dynamics and working relationships within your field of practice, and can interact effectively with colleagues and patients alike.

For the organisation, preceptorship is shown to have a positive impact on job satisfaction, which in turn improves retention and recruitment (NHS England, 2023a). The provision of preceptorship demonstrates a commitment to the well-being and progression of employees and leads to a more sustainable workforce, all of which helps to support service delivery and ultimately improve patient outcomes.

For the NQP, there is also a far more immediate benefit to a supportive preceptorship programme – definitive and direct assistance with the transition from being a student to autonomous practice. Kramer (1975) coined the term 'reality shock' to describe the conflict that newly qualified nurses experienced when comparing their ideological expectations of the role with the reality which faced them. The same emotional turbulence is experienced by NQPs, and the degree of difficulty you experience has a significant impact on both overall well-being and professional resilience (Phillips, 2024). Starting as an NQP is both a professional and a social transition, with the cumulative stressors of new clinical responsibilities combined with new employment. For many, it is also a transition from full-time education to full-time work. Health Education England's (2018) RePAIR report identified the impact of these factors on clinical confidence and highlighted the consequences of an unsupportive environment on both confidence and retention. Therefore, front-loaded clinical supervision as you start practising independently is crucial, and while this provision is an organisational rather than an individual requirement on which you may have little direct influence, it should be a significant factor when choosing which organisation to start your career journey in.

> 💬 **ADVICE**
>
> 'I started out treating my NQP portfolio as a tick box exercise — something I *had* to do in order to get by — but when I began using it as a guide for my CPD and focused on where I could actually develop, I got a lot more out of it.'

Preceptorship in Different Work Environments

For NQPs working outside the NHS, preceptorship may not be as readily available, or may take a different form. While not a requirement of registration, the Health and Care Professions Council (HCPC, 2023a) recently published its first *Principles of Preceptorship*, which highlight the benefits of such programmes and recommend the application of five key principles:

1. *Organisational culture and preceptorship*: ensuring a culture of learning which supports improvement while maintaining safe and effective patient care.

2. *Quality and oversight of preceptorship*: demonstrating the value of the health, well-being and confidence of registrants during times of transition.

3. *Preceptee empowerment*: enabling and inspiring new registrants to develop individual identity within a professional community.

4. *Preceptor role*: providing support for the supporters, with appropriate time, training and encouragement to act as professional role models.

5. *Delivering preceptorship programmes*: flexibility for individuals and organisations, but structured to deliver common themes.

The HCPC recommends that for paramedics working in environments that do not currently offer preceptorship, these principles can be used to make a business case for the development of such a scheme. This is applicable to private companies, voluntary or charitable organisations, and organisations delivering non-healthcare-related services.

Finally, although rare amongst NQPs, many paramedics work independently on a self-employed or subcontracted basis, and this can make access to preceptorship even more challenging. Establishing supportive links with other individuals and organisations is likely to be beneficial – in essence, a community of practice (Lave and Wenger, 1991) to connect those who are willing to provide preceptorship support with those who need it.

ADVICE

'Before accepting a new post, find out from the recruitment team what they offer in terms of preceptorship support.'

UK Ambulance Service Consolidation of Learning Programme

In December 2016, as part of the Urgent and Emergency Care Review,
paramedics in the English ambulance trusts were assimilated into a new
national job profile, providing greater consistency and transferability
between services (NHS Staff Council, 2016). At the same time, the role of
the NQP was created, alongside a national Consolidation of Learning Programme which was mandatory for all NQPs recruited to the English ambulance services after the 1st of September 2016. This two-year programme
was designed to provide structured support to integrate NQPs into
employment and offer time to consolidate the academic knowledge, skills
and experience gained as a student into confident independent practice
(NHS Employers, 2017) – in other words, a preceptorship programme.

Although every ambulance service is given autonomy to develop the
programme according to local needs and structure, there remains the
expectation that schemes are consistent with the national framework.
This has subsequently been supplemented by both the NHS England
(2023a) AHP Preceptorship Standards and Framework, and the HCPC
(2023a) Principles for Preceptorship.

Through the Consolidation of Learning Programme, employers are
expected to provide:

- Local induction
- Clinical supervision and mentorship

- Formal progress reviews every six months
- Individual development plans and learning opportunities, with constructive feedback
- Access to clinical decision-making support at all times
- Health and well-being support.

There are also responsibilities placed on the NQP, many of which align with the expectations of a registered clinician:

- Reflect on clinical practice and behaviours, and seek guidance when needed
- Maintain positive learning relationships and be open to constructive feedback
- Behave as ambassadors for the trust and demonstrate trust values
- Be prepared to raise constructive concerns and exercise the duty of candour
- Take ownership of the personal learning journey and engage with CPD opportunities
- Work within scope of practice and professional competency limits
- Maintain a practice portfolio to demonstrate competence against programme themes.

While the Consolidation of Learning Programme is only mandated within NHS ambulance trusts, several other organisations who employ NQPs have elected to adopt the same principles and thematic outcomes. It therefore offers a consistent and supportive approach which is portable between employers, and even where not mandated allows you to evidence professional development in a meaningful way, but with sufficient flexibility to meet individual needs. For this reason, activities in this book are designed to align to the learning outcomes of this, and any other, programme.

💬 ADVICE

'Like many tasks, I found that little and often was the best way to complete my portfolio – that way it felt less onerous, and I could focus on the parts that benefited me the most.'

Chapter 3
Regulation and Registration

In 1947, Jackie Robinson became the first black player in major league baseball when he joined the Brooklyn Dodgers and broke the colour barrier in a sport which had historically been segregated. He faced intense hostility from the outset, experiencing racial slurs, threats and aggressive tactics from players and fans alike. The team's manager, Branch Rickey, knew when he made the appointment that Robinson would face these challenges and gave a single clear instruction – that for the first two years, Robinson should not retaliate, no matter what abuse he suffered. Demonstrating this discipline was not about passivity or tolerance, but was a tactical decision which let Robinson's talent and professionalism speak for themselves, rather than becoming secondary to the prejudiced agenda of narrow-minded bigots (Povich, 1997).

Robinson honoured this commitment to restraint, and in doing so earned widespread respect, including the 'Rookie of the Year' title. His success set the stage for desegregation in baseball and, in part, the Civil Rights Movement. For Robinson, disciplined professionalism not only allowed him to excel in his career, but also served as a powerful, visible challenge to racial prejudice, showing millions of people that a professional response is a powerful driver for social change. Professionalism in healthcare may be less overt, but the individual and cultural impact are prodigious.

What It Means to be a Registered Professional

The term 'professionalism' is commonly used to describe a collection of behaviours, attitudes and values which define or identify a specific group. Although many individuals can articulate why they describe themselves as a professional, the concept itself has proven hard to define and is the subject of much academic debate. Within the field of medicine, there is no singularly accepted definition of what it means to be a professional. There are, however, a number of principles which are generally accepted as required in a professional (Birden et al., 2014):

- A code of conduct, which is developed and adopted by those within the profession
- A degree of status amongst the community in which they practise
- A body of evidence developed within the profession through which excellence in practice is maintained
- Accountability, underpinned by self-regulation and trustworthiness
- Altruism, prioritising the needs of the people for whom the professional is responsible.

While many will consider these principles reasonable, they are far from simple – nor are they uncontested. Disagreements often stem from the simple definition of 'good', particularly within the field of ethics. For example, if you spend an extended period of time with one patient, are you promoting that person's best interests or neglecting other patients who may be waiting for help? Or if you transport a patient to a more remote hospital for humanitarian reasons, are you supporting patient-centred care or threatening the sustainability of an already challenged healthcare system? As is frequently the case with ethical dilemmas, there is no clear correct answer. Challenge also arises regarding the extent to which selflessness should be applied – short-term hardships such as delayed breaks or having to work nightshifts can be accepted, but many NQPs struggle with the degree to which they should put themselves at risk to support others, particularly when balancing a duty of care with self-preservation. Over the past 20 years, several high-profile inquests have promoted the importance of emergency services workers accepting a degree of risk when providing unplanned care (Pollock, 2013), but this can be difficult to reconcile with maintaining personal safety.

There is one further expectation which is common amongst many other professions: discipline. For pilots, professional athletes, police and others, upholding discipline is a core component of their professional identity. Conversely, in medicine the need for discipline is rejected in favour of autonomy, a principle which could be considered the antithesis of such control (Gawunde, 2009). Despite being hard to apply, particularly within a field which perniciously promotes self-sufficiency and independent decision making as ideals, a disciplined approach which prioritises consistency over individual choice can be an effective safety mechanism for the NQP. While still developing your bank of experience on which decisions are based, the consistent application of evidence-based guidelines and professional codes of conduct offers a safe model of care on which to develop your future expertise.

> ### ✎ ACTIVITY
>
> Imagine you are a patient needing treatment. What expectations would you have of the person who comes to your aid? Now think what you can do in your own practice to ensure these expectations are met.

The Role of the HCPC

Within the UK, the Health Professions Order 2001 protects the title 'paramedic' and makes it a legal requirement for anybody practising under this title to be registered with the HCPC.

The overarching role of the HCPC is to protect the public, through the regulation of 15 health and care professions within the UK, including paramedics. Registration with the HCPC is a requirement of practice as a paramedic, and provides professional credibility and public assurance. This is achieved through three main areas of work.

Set Standards for Education and Approve Programmes

The HCPC reviews organisations that deliver paramedic programmes of education, and approves these based on its published Standards of Education and Training (SET). These define the level of qualification required for entry onto the register. Since 2021 this has required a

Bachelor's degree with honours, alongside admission requirements, programme design (including the requirement for practice-based learning), quality assurance and assessment methodologies.

The HCPC maintains a list of approved programmes on its website and can support individuals who raise concerns about these, although it does encourage a local resolution to be attempted first.

Maintaining the Register

The HCPC maintains a public register of all HCPs who maintain their standards of training, skills and health to be able to practise safely. It allows both patients and employers to verify professional registration status, and includes annotations relating to additional rights (such as supplementary and independent prescribing), as well as identifying if a registrant is currently subject to any restrictions in their practice.

All paramedics are required to renew registration every two years, which involves making a professional declaration that they are continuing to practise and meet the requirements of registration.

Managing Fitness to Practise Concerns

Where there is a risk that a paramedic's ability to practise safely is impaired, the HCPC will investigate the matter and, where deemed necessary, apply sanctions. While this is often a cause of anxiety for NQPs, the process is essential for maintaining public trust and ensuring that all professionals deliver safe, high-quality care. Most paramedics will never experience this. Further information is provided in Chapter 7.

Gaining HCPC Registration

As implied by the title of 'registration', the HCPC maintains a register of all paramedics currently authorised to practise under that title in the UK – currently over 40,000 in total (HCPC, 2025). This is not an automatic process, and to be added to the register, after successfully completing appropriate professional training, you must apply to the HCPC. For most applicants, this will involve completing an online form and waiting for your university to confirm to the HCPC that an approved qualification was successfully achieved (sometimes referred to as a 'pass list').

The application form itself involves a number of stages:

- Confirming you have read key documents, particularly the *Standards of Proficiency for Paramedics* and the *Standards of Conduct, Performance and Ethics*

- Providing personal details, both for administrative purposes and to confirm identity, which is completed by providing certified copies of an identity document

- Completing character and health declarations to indicate that there are no concerns around current fitness to practise

- Identifying the approved education programme undertaken to qualify as a paramedic

- Final declarations, which act as your electronic signature to confirm the information provided is accurate

- Optional Equality, Diversity and Inclusion (EDI) monitoring data to complete, which are recorded separately from the application and are used anonymously to support the HCPC in meeting legal and ethical equality standards.

You will need to pay a registration fee once qualification status has been confirmed. After the fee has been paid, registration will be confirmed by email within a few days and your new registration number, prefixed 'PA', will be issued. This is the unique identifier used to verify registration and will usually be requested by employers.

> 💬 **ADVICE**
>
> 'When applying for registration, use your own email address – I used my university email which I then lost access to having completed the course, which made things more stressful than they needed to be!'

Specific Circumstances

There are some circumstances in which the application process will be slightly different, for example:

- If you apply from outside of the UK or you have not completed an approved qualification in the past five years, you will need to provide evidence that your training and qualification match those required by the HCPC.

- If you are returning to the register having previously lapsed your registration, you may need to provide evidence of currency and a suitable return to practice programme.

- If you have character or health concerns which may affect your ability to practise safely, you will have to provide further details to be reviewed by a panel.

While each of these circumstances can prolong the time it takes for registration to be obtained, there is plenty of information on the HCPC website and through online forums to support you through this process. Often, your employer may also be able to provide help and advice.

💬 ADVICE

'Even if you are delayed starting employment for any reason, it is better to register with the HCPC as soon as eligible to do so. This ensures you receive any relevant communications and can legally use the title of paramedic.'

✏️ ACTIVITY

One of the expectations of a registered paramedic is to understand and adhere to the HCPC standards. Take the opportunity to read through these and reflect on how you can ensure you apply them consistently.

Professional Standards and Behaviour

The professionalisation of paramedicine is a relatively recent, and ongoing, process. Developing from the 'extended skills' training provided to select ambulance personnel in the 1970s, the early role of the paramedic was to provide more advanced care on scene – a dramatic shift from the transport-focused approach of the time. Early training focused on critical care and life-saving interventions but changes in industry, improvements in safety and a significant shift in the demand profile and nature of work undertaken by ambulance services mean that this is now the minority of patient presentations seen by paramedics, and the profession has had to evolve even while becoming established (Newton, 2012).

It was only in the late 1990s that undergraduate paramedic degrees were first introduced, changing the nature of paramedic education and prioritising underpinning knowledge and critical reasoning over 'skills and drills'. In 2000 state registration became a mandatory requirement, introducing for the first time a consistent code of conduct to which all paramedics were required to subscribe (College of Paramedics, 2021).

Higher education and registration, coupled with the shift in demand towards acute and urgent care, paved the way for diversification in paramedicine, and has resulted in the vast range of employment opportunities now available for paramedics. The pace of professionalisation has not been without problems, however, requiring a paradigm shift in the culture of ambulance services – a shift which is still ongoing, with several areas still requiring improvement despite the progress which has been made to date (Melia, 2024).

As you first enter the profession, adoption of the professional standards required by the HCPC (2024) can seem daunting. Although you will have gained some familiarity through the published guidance on conduct and ethics for students (HCPC, 2024), lived experience often varies, which can lead to a disconnect between the professional expectations taught, and those which are role-modelled by others and therefore adopted into your individual practice. The factors which promote and inhibit professionalism are varied, and maintaining it requires employer and regulator involvement alongside individual behaviours and values.

When thinking about practical application, there are two primary considerations. First, to acknowledge that professionalism is intrinsically linked to identity as much as to behaviour (First et al., 2012) – and perhaps the key to professionalism is to recognise yourself as a professional, rather than solely a clinician. The second is that demonstrating professional standards is as much about the behaviour of others as that of yourself, as summarised by David Morrison (Osborne, 2015) – 'the standard you walk past is the standard you accept'.

✍ ACTIVITY

Create a spreadsheet which lists the HCPC *Standards of Proficiency for Paramedics*. Every time you undertake any activity which develops or maintains a standard, make a note within the spreadsheet to demonstrate ongoing adherence to the standards.

Scope of Practice

The term 'scope of practice' (SOP) is generally used to refer to the limit of an individual's knowledge, skill and experience in the context of their professional activity, ensuring they can practise safely and lawfully within their current role (Downie et al., 2023). Although the SOP for all NQPs is likely to be similar, there are variations between employers in terms of what you are both expected and permitted to do, which is influenced by the working environment, nature of care provided, education and supervision, and organisational preference.

Specific SOP will be determined by your employer and is subject to the clinical governance processes and professional indemnity arrangements in place. For self-employed practitioners, the latter of these is significant – where most NQPs would be insured for their acts and omissions through their employer, self-employed individuals are required to maintain their own indemnity cover.

It is important that you are both aware of, and adhere to, your SOP. For an inexperienced practitioner, this can present challenges, particularly in terms of recognising the limitations of your role. Gaining experience involves consolidating theoretical knowledge and applying it to novel situations, often with a degree of urgency and a perception of limited support. When determining whether to undertake a particular action, it can be helpful to apply the four questions in Figure 3.1, which highlight two intrinsic and two extrinsic factors to identify SOP.

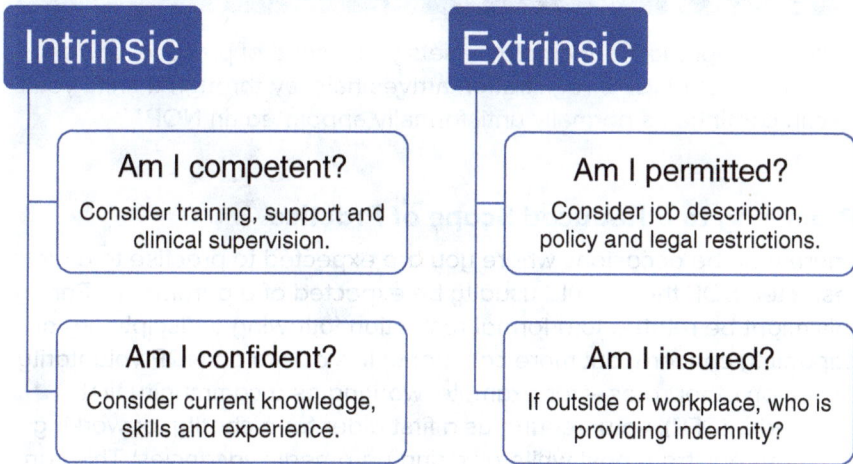

Intrinsic

Am I competent?
Consider training, support and clinical supervision.

Am I confident?
Consider current knowledge, skills and experience.

Extrinsic

Am I permitted?
Consider job description, policy and legal restrictions.

Am I insured?
If outside of workplace, who is providing indemnity?

Figure 3.1 – Is it in my scope?

✏️ ACTIVITY

Consider a situation (either from experience or a hypothetical case study) where you reach the limit of your scope of practice. Consider how you could apply the questions in Figure 3.1 to ensure you continue to practise safely.

For most paramedics, SOP will change throughout your career. The HCPC (2023b) *Standards of Proficiency for Paramedics* provide a clear outline of what is expected, but with increasing opportunities for specialisation or non-patient-facing roles, you may find that your SOP narrows and you no longer demonstrate every standard, or do so in a different way than you did previously. Fundamentally, as long as you continue to make informed, reasoned decisions to ensure your actions safeguard the well-being of service users, and do not directly breach the standards of proficiency (as opposed to failing to demonstrate them), your SOP is unlikely to be a cause for concern.

> ### 💬 ADVICE
>
> 'Remember that your employer sets your scope of practice, so don't panic if your HCPC registration arrives halfway through a shift; you can continue as normally until formally appointed an NQP.'

Practising to a Reduced Scope of Practice

There may be occasions where you are expected to practise to a more restricted SOP than would usually be expected of a paramedic. Rarely, this might be related to a formal restriction following a disciplinary or capability concern, but more commonly it is due to an NQP voluntarily taking on other roles – for example, working as a community first responder (CFR), volunteering as a first aider for a charity, or working in a non-registrant post while awaiting paramedic vacancies. This can cause concern around balancing the limitations of these roles with the expectations of the HCPC, but as long as you continue to practise safely within the limits of your designated role, and do not breach any HCPC standards, this would not cause any problems with your fitness to practise (HCPC and College of Paramedics, 2020).

If circumstances arose where a patient required care or interventions that you were able to provide but that were outside the SOP for the role you were undertaking, you would be expected to seek further assistance (including calling 999 if necessary), or use your professional judgement to act appropriately and in the best interests of the patient.

Recognising Limitations

At the point of registration, you are likely to have a sound, up-to-date theoretical knowledge on which to base your clinical practice, with significant research, critical analysis and reflection having been instilled in you during your programme of education. Clinical skills will have been regularly practised, supervised, perfected and assessed, and while this may not be reflected in your confidence, you can take reassurance from the fact that, academically at least, you are amongst the most current clinicians in practice – at least until the next cohort graduates.

This can, in some cases, lead to a misplaced sense of capability, particularly when faced with situations in independent practice which have been studied but not yet experienced. The application of knowledge can be nuanced, and the increased gravity of a patient with genuine health concerns coupled with the perceived external pressure which comes with registration can accentuate any small knowledge gaps but can also sometimes lead to these being masked. Acknowledging this theory–practice divide and associated limitations is essential to maintain safe practice and minimise risk.

Limitations may manifest in various forms: gaps in knowledge about certain conditions, uncertainty in managing complex cases, or lack of confidence in performing clinical procedures. These are natural challenges which come with inexperience, but recognising these boundaries supports a realistic awareness of your capability and reduces the risk of errors that may compromise patient safety. It also fosters humility and provides a foundation for a career based on professional accountability and continuous learning.

Acknowledging personal limitation can be emotionally taxing and professionally uncomfortable at times, particularly in a high-stakes environment where patient outcomes are affected by clinician expertise. Historically, the public perception of healthcare is one of unwavering accuracy (consider phrases such as 'doctor knows best'), and this can produce an environment where self-doubt prevails but remains concealed. Being open, while challenging, supports a safe culture of resilience where opportunities for learning are celebrated over expectations of infallibility, and is key in cultivating a growth, rather than a fixed, mindset (Dweck, 2017). Adopting a growth mindset profoundly influences how you view suboptimal performance, and recognising limitations as opportunities rather than deficits will ultimately benefit both you and the patient.

As the philosopher Maimonides recognised, perfection of the art of medicine takes longer than the human lifespan affords (Desveaux and Ivers, 2024), and it is therefore important for all clinicians to accept the inevitability of limitation.

> ### ✏️ ACTIVITY
>
> Do you undertake clinical practice or strive for clinical perfection? Make a list of the risks and benefits of each approach and compare these to your personal mindset.

The College of Paramedics

First founded in 2001 as the British Paramedic Association, the College of Paramedics (name adopted in 2004) is the professional body for all paramedics working in the UK, striving to promote and develop the paramedic profession. The College represents its members in any matter which affects clinical practice, and publishes a range of documents which underpin the profession, including undergraduate and postgraduate curricula, a career framework, and guidance and position statements. It holds a strategic role in shaping policy and frequently speaks on behalf of and in support of the profession in legislative, political and media settings.

As a professional body, the College of Paramedics is distinct from the HCPC (which is the regulator) but often engages with the HCPC and other stakeholders as one of the 'professional, statutory or regulatory bodies' (PSRB), which is an umbrella term for the diverse groups which have a degree of authority over a profession.

In 2024, the College was granted a Royal Charter in recognition of its objectives to inspire and enable all paramedics to participate in the profession within an environment based on safety, collegiality, inclusiveness, mental and physical well-being and innovation. Membership of the College is open to all registered paramedics within the UK, as well as students working towards this status and other interested supporters. More information is available from the College of Paramedics website. As an NQP, membership offers you personal benefits (including educational opportunities, discounts and legal support) as well as the representation at a national level of the profession, education and careers of paramedics.

> ### 💬 ADVICE
>
> 'Joining the College of Paramedics felt like a natural step to support my profession, and I was even able to claim tax relief on the membership subscription!'

Chapter 4
Clinical Practice

In the mid-19th century, maternal mortality rates were high, particularly within hospitals. A Hungarian physician, Ignaz Semmelweis, noticed starkly higher death rates in mothers attended to by doctors compared to those with midwife-led deliveries, and discovered that unlike midwives, doctors frequently came directly from performing autopsies to undertake deliveries. He hypothesised that 'cadaverous particles' were being transferred from corpses to patients, causing infection, and instituted a simple, but novel, practice of handwashing before delivering babies. To the astonishment of colleagues, death rates dramatically decreased but the practice was widely rejected by doctors who were offended by the implication that they were causing harm (Best and Neuhauser, 2004). It wasn't until decades later that the universally accepted, evidence-based practice of hand hygiene became embedded in medicine, and in the interim patients continued to die simply due to a failure to meet the most basic of patient expectations and consider the evidence.

Patient Expectations

Ensuring you have a good understanding of patient expectations supports the delivery of high-quality patient care. Patients often experience anxiety or fear when seeking healthcare, caused by the effect of the illness or injury and exacerbated by the experience of being dependent on others for help. Situations which are an everyday occurrence for paramedics are often a once in a lifetime event for the patient – a form of experience asymmetry, where perceptions of a singular event vary based on differing prior experience. It can be helpful to consider this when dealing with incidents which are considered routine or mundane, as it encourages greater consideration of the patient perspective.

What constitutes a timely response will vary by working environment, and despite a greater emphasis on clinical prioritisation, pressures within healthcare services often result in long waiting times for patients. This can be challenging, as waiting times are largely outside your control, but awareness of this expectation can influence your initial communication with the patient (particularly where attendance has been delayed) and therefore defuse, rather than escalate, any potential tensions.

Research commissioned by the Care Quality Commission (CQC, 2015) aimed to identify what constituted outstanding patient care and while the results are unsurprising, they provide key areas of focus for the NQP:

- Immediate recognition of urgent situations
- Clear, professional communication
- Dignity and respect
- Comfort and reassurance
- Personalised care
- A resolution to clinical needs (including transport where appropriate).

Unlike response times, each of these can be directly influenced by your approach, leading to a positive impact on the patient experience. A common cause of frustration is where the patient expectation does not align with that of the clinician – this can often be resolved by communication and directly asking the patient key questions using the ECHO mnemonic. What are their:

- **E**xpectations
- **C**oncerns
- **H**opes
- **O**utcome desired?

Consider a situation where the concerns and expectations of a patient have differed from your own. How did this impact on your communication with the patient? How do you ensure your communication remains professional where there is disagreement?

Duty of Care

A duty of care is an obligation placed on people to act in a certain way towards others, and exists for NQPs as a moral, professional and legal imperative. The moral aspect stems largely from societal expectations and is a matter for individual conscience – most individuals who choose to work in healthcare do so with the desire to help others.

Professional duty of care exists through your employment contract, which usually references organisational policies and procedures to guide expectations around standards of care. As a registrant, you also have a professional duty through your regulatory body.

Although legal jurisdiction varies slightly between the devolved nations of the UK, duty of care principles remain largely consistent. Article 2 of the Human Rights Act 1998 introduces an active duty on public sector organisations to do everything that can reasonably be done to protect individuals who are at immediate risk – either where this risk is known or should be known (Van Colle v CC of Hertfordshire [2007] EWCA Civ 325). There are, however, exceptions to this – clinicians are not expected to sacrifice their own life to save someone else. Additionally, unlike the police and fire services, the NHS Ambulance Service has a legal duty to provide a reasonable standard of care to patients without unreasonable delay – with effect from when the service accepts the call (Kent v Griffiths [2001] QB 36). Care is defined as being of a reasonable standard when it is supported by a responsible body of medical opinion (Bolam v Friern Hospital Management Committee [1957] 2 All ER 118). Any departure from these expectations could be considered negligence, and while the established duty of care specifically applies to NHS Ambulance Services, it is likely that the same principles could be applied to paramedics working in other environments.

> ### ✍ ACTIVITY
>
> Consider how you can ensure that your practice as an NQP meets the established duty of care from a moral, professional and legal perspective. What are the personal and professional risks of failing to meet these obligations?

The professional and legal duty of care only applies within the workplace setting and you are under no obligation to volunteer assistance in an emergency situation that arises outside work, since you have not assumed responsibility for that patient. If, however, you choose to help then there is an expectation that the standard of care would be reasonable – in other words, the fact that the care is provided voluntarily and outside work would not excuse errors in the care provided. You may also not be covered by liability insurance, although this does depend on the individual circumstances. The HCPC places no obligation on registrants to render aid when 'off duty', stating 'We do not treat actions as a "good Samaritan" – someone who provides first aid or other emergency help when there is no professional obligation to do so – as professional practice...' (HCPC, 2014).

Defensive Versus Defensible Practice

When providing care, NQPs are frequently faced with high-pressure situations that require quick decisions based on critical thinking and rapid action. Even with patients who are not time critical, NQPs work autonomously with minimal supervision and support, and it is therefore essential to distinguish between defensive and defensible care. Despite sounding similar, understanding the difference is crucial for practising safely and ethically while maintaining professional accountability.

Defensive care refers to actions you take that are primarily motivated through fear of legal consequences or professional criticism, rather than the best interests of the patient. This approach leads to unnecessary treatments, investigations or referrals aimed at managing the risk to the clinician. It is usually more time-consuming, and therapeutic benefits are often overshadowed by detriments to the holistic treatment of the patient, including unnecessary hospital visits, inconvenience, increased anxiety and repeat presentations.

Perhaps the most common example of defensive practice by NQPs is transporting patients to hospital instead of utilising appropriate alternative care pathways or community treatment options. The outdated adage 'nobody gets fired for taking their patient to hospital' is still presented as a clinical rationale, but even less extreme reasons such as a lack of familiarity with local pathways or anxiety around the risks of referring a patient still have the same outcome. Other examples of defensive practice include performing every test and examination available on patients with a simple or well-defined presentation, and overcautious safety net advice which encourages an unrequired follow-up attendance.

It is important to note that in isolation, none of the actions identified above is intrinsically harmful or inappropriate – hospital conveyance, thorough patient assessment and provision of worsening care advice are all good practice when part of a balanced patient management plan. Instead, it is when these approaches are used to avoid clinical decision making or for your own benefit that they become potentially harmful. Unintended consequences can include exposing the patient to iatrogenic harm through overtreatment or avoidable hospital attendance with the associated risks (such as healthcare-acquired infections), placing additional strain on already overburdened healthcare systems, and further reducing your confidence and ability.

ACTIVITY

Defensive practice focuses on risks to the clinician, whereas defensible practice considers the wider impact of decisions on the patient. Consider what mitigations you could utilise to reduce identified risks to an acceptable level.

In contrast, defensible care is grounded in clinical reasoning, professional guidelines and evidence-based practice. It requires you to make sound, well-documented decisions that prioritise patient welfare, even in complex or ambiguous situations. Any care provided is defendable because it follows established best practice, is supported by appropriate clinical judgement and the rationale for decisions is clearly recorded.

Defensible care emphasises the importance of critical thinking – in other words analysing the benefits and risks of each option before selecting the most appropriate based on the patient's unique circumstances. You must draw on your knowledge, skills and experience when making decisions, utilising other sources of information and support as appropriate – as your experience increases, the support requirement may change. Decisions should incorporate not only the immediate needs of the patient and the clinical assessment, but also the broader ethical, legal and holistic considerations. In doing so, even if an adverse event occurs, the decision will be defensible by showing that the care was provided in line with the evidence base, patient wishes and sound clinical judgement.

Documentation: The Key to Defensible Practice

One of the most important aspects of delivering defensible care is accurate and thorough documentation. Although methodology varies by organisation, clear documentation helps demonstrate that clinical decisions were based on objective assessment, relevant patient information and professional guidelines. As well as supporting the ongoing care of the patient, it provides a record that can be referred to if your decisions are ever challenged.

Clinical records should generally adhere to the following principles:

- **Contemporaneous:** made at the time of the patient encounter, or as soon afterwards as possible (clearly timed and dated).

- **Clear:** legible (if handwritten) and unambiguous in terms of the language used. Avoid abbreviations and colloquialisms (slang terms).

- **C**oncise: only record pertinent information and avoid extended but unnecessary narrative. Where recording decisions, include all options considered, and the rationale for the chosen approach.

- **C**omplete: ensure the key details are included; organisations may have a 'minimum data set' which must be included on every record.

- **C**onsistent and factual: focus on facts rather than subjective opinions.

- **C**orrect: if information is incomplete or unavailable, record why. Check following completion and correct any errors.

- **C**onfidential: completed patient records are sensitive personal data.

✏️ ACTIVITY

Obtain redacted copies of a selection of patient records that you have completed recently and undertake a personal audit. How well do they comply with the principles above? Highlight any parts which do not comply (irrelevant information, opinion, missed information). Consider what influences the quality of your patient records and how this could be improved.

Evidence-based Practice

In the 1950s, the development of synthetic medications was a novel concept, with limited governance or scientific oversight and significant opportunities for financial reward. Against this background a new 'wonder drug' emerged, a chemically simple product with minimal identified side-effects which provided antiemetic treatment for a prevalent, and sometimes debilitating, condition. The drug was called thalidomide (Ridings, 2013).

The rapidity with which the drug was accepted and prescribed is an indictment of the way in which medicine was practised at the time, but paved the way for a seminal paper by J. R. Hampton (1983) in which he debated the concept of what is now known as evidence-based practice (EBP).

For NQPs today, the concept of providing treatment without a cogent evidence base is almost incomprehensible, with paramedic education increasingly focused on the underpinning research for assessment methodology and interventions. Despite the wealth of scientific literature on which current clinical practice is based, it is common for this to have its roots in other disciplines and while the general principles may be applicable to paramedicine, it is important to maintain a discerning approach.

You may therefore find that it is the abundance of available literature, rather than any scarcity, which poses the biggest challenge. Clinical practice guidelines, such as those supplied by the Joint Royal Colleges Ambulance Liaison Committee (JRCALC), offer a consensus opinion which provides a safe standard of care to patients, even where there may be isolated or specific cases which would benefit from an alternative approach. Bodies such as the National Institute for Health and Care Excellence (NICE, 2018) offer principles for putting evidence-based guidance into practice, but these are focused on organisational development rather than individual clinical practice.

The ongoing flow of knowledge can feel overwhelming, as you are faced with a daily onslaught of facts, opinions, data, recommendations and rumours all posing as useful information. Add to this that information is often shared through the filter of another individual's interpretation, and it can be difficult to know where to start. The statement 'Everything we hear is an opinion, not a fact. Everything we see is a perspective, not the truth' is commonly attributed to the philosopher Marcus Aurelius, but when making decisions which affect patient outcomes, there is an understandable desire for something more definitive than opinion and perspective.

There are various models for using EBP in a range of settings, but the methodology remains broadly consistent. The following approach, adapted from Titler (2006), provides a step-wise process which can be applied at the point of care.

1. *Ask* the question: converting the clinical situation or problem into a question which can be answered.

2. *Acquire* best evidence: using a systematic process to gather information from available sources.

3. *Appraise* the information: critically judge the validity (trustworthiness) and relevance (usefulness).

4. *Aggregate* sources: balance and combine the information from different sources, attaching appropriate weight to each source.

5. *Apply* the evidence: incorporate the outcome reached into the decision-making process and direct patient care.

6. *Assess* the outcome: consider the results of the decision to influence future decisions for the same patient, and guide reflection for future patients.

The source of evidence will vary depending on the circumstances in which it is being applied. Although expert opinion is generally considered the weakest form of evidence (Greenhalgh, 2010), at the point of care it may be all that is directly available to support your decision making. Despite critics arguing that it may not lead to the best possible care for all patients, this is where the use of published clinical practice guidelines by NQPs offers a major advantage by presenting EBP for frequently seen patient presentations in an accessible and easily referenced format. Many organisations, including those adopting the National Ambulance Service NQP programme, restrict NQPs from deviating from these approved guidelines without the authorisation of an experienced clinician, which provides a safety net for both you and the patient while still allowing for autonomous practice and the use of alternative evidence sources.

ACTIVITY

Consider what sources of information you might use to provide the evidence base for your own practice. How can you simply and safely risk assess these to ensure they benefit patient care? How would you ensure the accuracy of information you share with others?

> ### 💬 ADVICE
>
> 'At university I was taught about the risks of sticking rigidly to the JRCALC guidelines, but the more I studied, the more I became aware of differences in opinion and conflicting research, which makes the evidence base in JRCALC feel much more appealing!'

Requesting and Utilising Additional Support

In clinical practice, there will be occasions when you are faced with a situation which exceeds the scope of your expertise or the available resources. While this situation is not exclusive to NQPs, it is logical to expect an inexperienced practitioner to require support more frequently than veteran colleagues, although this should not be considered a shortfall in ability. Knowing how and when to ask for help is an essential quality for all working in a healthcare setting. The reason for, and nature of, support required may vary – some of the more common reasons are considered below. It is important to be aware that the availability, and method of requesting, additional help vary considerably between organisations – identifying the local options is an important part of organisational induction and there is no harm in seeking clarity if unsure.

Reasons for Requesting Support

Severe or deteriorating patients

Critically ill, haemodynamically unstable or rapidly deteriorating patients will probably benefit from having additional experienced or specialist clinicians on scene. This may be due to the volume of interventions required (for example, a cardiac arrest requires multiple concurrent actions by attending clinicians), the rarity of the presentation (major trauma is seen infrequently by ambulance clinicians) or the need for interventions learned during education but never practised independently (skills fade in such circumstances is common) (Henderson et al., 2019).

Specialist conditions

This doesn't solely refer to high-acuity presentations, such as complications of childbirth, but can include presentations which are either unusual or fall outside the usual scope of paramedics. In such circumstances, either seeking remote support on scene or referring the patient to an appropriate specialist service can ensure the patient receives a high standard of care and management of the clinical risk.

Multiple casualties

This can range from incidental secondary patients to major incidents. Although the latter is rare, promptly requesting additional resources is recommended – it is usually easier to scale down the response at a later stage than to continuously increase it. Ensure familiarity with organisational policies for large-scale incidents, and consider referring to the Joint Emergency Services Interoperability Programme (JESIP) to ensure partnership working at multi-agency incidents (JESIP, 2024).

High-risk decisions

These are not always decisions which need to be made rapidly, but those which have the potential for long-term patient harm or even death if the wrong decision is made. Best practice involves sharing the decision with another qualified person, and some organisations mandate this for NQPs for high-risk decisions.

Unfamiliar situations

Limited experience leads to a greater likelihood of encountering situations which are novel to the clinician. While your confidence and competence continue to develop, seeking guidance from others can ensure clinical safety and act as a valuable learning opportunity.

Gaining and Maintaining Clinical Confidence

Transitioning from the role of student to practising clinician can feel overwhelming at times. Moving from a supervised learning environment to taking full responsibility for patient care can challenge the confidence of even the strongest learner. When comparing the inexperience you felt as a brand new student paramedic on your first day to the significant developments that have allowed you to successfully complete the course and register as a paramedic, it can be even more difficult to return to being a novice (albeit as a novice qualified paramedic rather than a novice student). Lack of confidence often stems from self-imposed pressure rather than any external expectation, with NQPs focusing more on the 'qualified' element of their job title than the 'newly' part. Add to this the fact that it is only recently that NQPs have been distinguished from their experienced colleagues and recognition of the differentiated support required by inexperienced practitioners remains variable, and it is unsurprising that many NQPs will experience a crisis in confidence when they move into registered practice.

The term 'imposter syndrome' was first used in 1978 to describe the persistent feeling of self-doubt or inadequacy stemming from individuals believing they are not as competent as others perceive or expect them to be (Clance and Imes, 1978). Imposter syndrome is prevalent amongst HCPs (Health Education England, 2021), and although commonly associated with being newly qualified, it can occur at all grades and experience levels, often when moving into new working environments or dealing with unfamiliar situations. If left unchecked, it can undermine confidence and adversely affect job performance but with the right strategies, it is possible to overcome these negative feelings (Bandali, 2022).

The first step in overcoming imposter syndrome is to recognise that it exists. When experiencing feelings of self-doubt, it is easy to forget how prevalent this is or to perceive that your uncertainty is more pronounced or 'worse' than that of your peers. Acknowledging the feelings as a psychological phenomenon, rather than a true reflection of your ability, is crucial (Bravata et al., 2020). Once recognised, it becomes easier to argue against any resulting negative thoughts that arise – for example, by reframing doubts into positive affirmations, similar to undertaking a critical appraisal of an evidence base (Dweck, 2017). This also requires acceptance that perfection is unrealistic and mistakes are inevitable – making a mistake is not a sign of failure, but failing to learn from such situations would be a mistake.

Rather than fearing failure, view it as an opportunity to improve, but remain equally conscious of your achievements and celebrate these (Howlett, 2019). Reflect on outcomes and ensure the focus remains on individual achievement, rather than the effect this has had on others. While this may feel egocentric, it helps to reinforce personal validation, rather than linking self-worth to the views of others. Finally, be willing to ask for help – open and honest communication can both be reassuring and offer valuable feedback. Sometimes, simply hearing that others have felt the same way you do can be a powerful relief.

Using this approach (Figure 4.1) will not necessarily solve imposter syndrome, and many excellent clinicians go on to experience the effects at different stages throughout their career. It can, however, help individuals who are prone to questioning their achievements to feel more confident in their clinical practice and push themselves to develop.

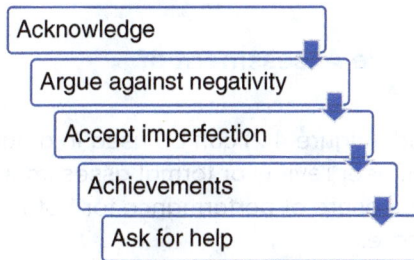

Acknowledge

Argue against negativity

Accept imperfection

Achievements

Ask for help

Figure 4.1 – Dealing with imposter syndrome.

💬 ADVICE

'The biggest difference I have noticed as I have gained experience is not that I feel better prepared to deal with every situation, but that I feel more confident that I will be able to manage any situation for long enough for help to get to me, or me to get the patient to further help.'

Measuring and Recording Clinical Performance

A key to ensuring development as a clinician is being able to objectively review and record clinical performance. There are numerous tools and frameworks available to support with this to varying degrees of complexity, but using a consistent approach over an extended period can be helpful to identify trends and highlight areas for improvement. The minimum goal of any clinician should be to remain competent and confident in all areas of practice, striving for professional development, while also acknowledging that there can be periods of time or areas of focus where this is not maintained. Recording a snapshot of performance at specific moments allows for progress tracking, identification of training needs and setting development goals. This not only enhances your performance but also ensures that you continue to deliver safe, effective care while diversifying your career (Eaton, 2023).

Structured Objective Assessment of Performance (SOAP)

The SOAP framework (Figure 4.2) can be used in a number of ways – individual reflection, peer review or formal assessment. It is designed to be applied as a measure of performance for both non-clinical and clinical aspects of care.

✏️ ACTIVITY

Consider how you could use the SOAP framework to review and reflect on your clinical practice. How might this change as your experience increases?

OBJECTIVE

Clinicians should be competent and confident to work to their current scope of practice

Clinical competence

R — **Remedial action**
Unable to work to current scope of practice without additional training, support, or clinical supervision

I — **Improvement needed**
Generally able to work at current scope however would benefit from further support to work independently

C — **Competent**
Works to a consistently safe standard and able to work to current scope of practice without additional support

E — **Excellent**
Consistently exceeds standard required whilst practicing safely within current scope of practice

Professional confidence

A — **Anxious**
Lacks confidence in own ability leading to difficulty with decision-making and affecting personal wellbeing

C — **Confident**
Able to practice independently as appropriate for scope of practice, but seeks support when required

E — **Extremely confident**
Highly independent and assured of own ability - may be appropriate but may be misplaced (arrogance)

Consider:
- Formal Education Referral
- Individual action plan
- Clinical supervision
- Practice education support
- Training Needs Analysis

Requires support

Requires development

Consider:
- Career conversation
- Appraisal
- Clinical supervision
- Development opportunities

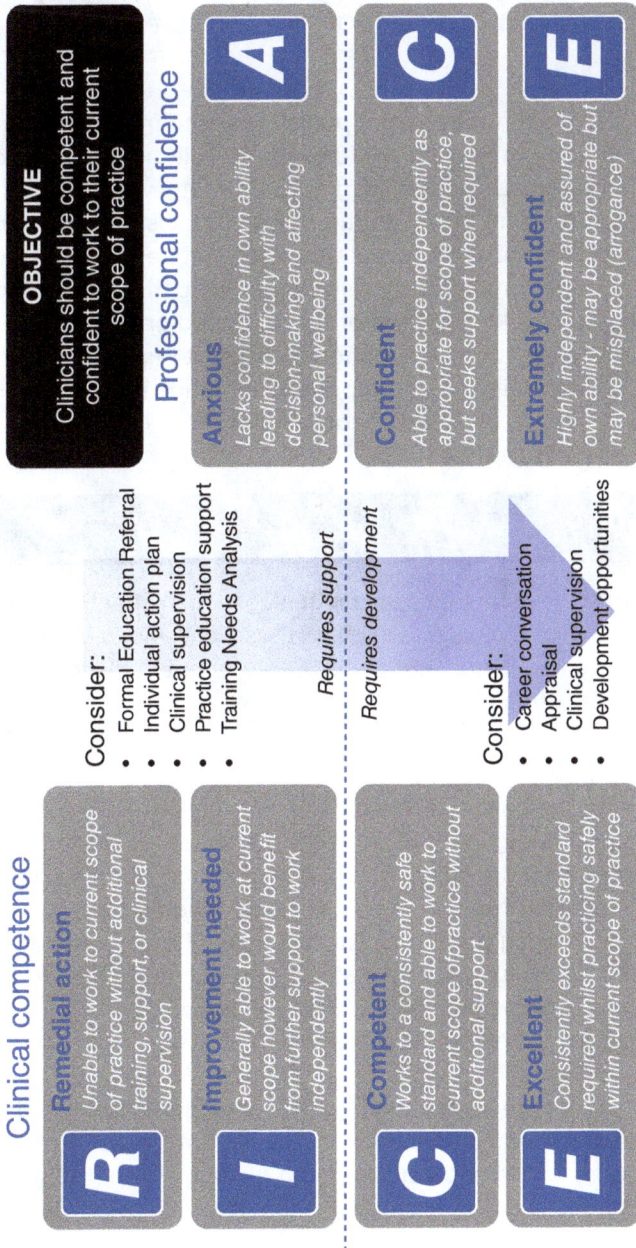

Figure 4.2 – Structured Objective Assessment of Performance.

Clinical Decision Making as an Inexperienced Practitioner

Making decisions is a fundamental part of life, and from an early age you have learned to process the information available (input) and reach a conclusion (output). Decisions vary in complexity, volume and impact, and although there may be similarities, no two decisions are identical since later decisions can incorporate the experiences gained through making earlier decisions. Clinical decision making involves balancing the information about known best practice (based on evidence and guidelines), awareness of the situation or context (based on your experience) and knowledge of the patient condition (obtained through patient assessment), to reach a suitable outcome.

ACTIVITY

How many different factors can you think of which affect your clinical decision making? Consider which of these are within your control and which are not. What safeguards can you put in place to ensure your decisions remain safe?

Decision making takes place on a spectrum from rapid and intuitive to measured and analytical. You make thousands of decisions every day, not solely related to clinical care but also operational, logistical, resource management and personal needs. Many of these will be simple, high-frequency decisions with a low level of uncertainty and can be made intuitively using heuristics – mental shortcuts founded in generalisations and experience. This same approach can be applied to more complex decisions but requires experience to be effective.

Recognition-primed decision making (RPD) is frequently utilised by paramedics, where similarities between cases can be used as a cognitive bypass to make a safe decision quickly (Klein, 1998). There are two difficulties with this – the first is that it relies on previous exposure to similar circumstances, and the second is that you must be able to contextualise those circumstances to the current situation. Both rely on having significant experience and since experience is an attribute which can only be gained over time, NQPs often rely on more cognitive processes of decision making. Reassuringly, however, experience has not been shown to improve the quality of decision making (Kirkebøen, 2009) – only the speed and method through which a decision is made, and confidence in making that decision.

Decision-making Competencies

Decision making is not solely based on experience, and there are several core skills which can support effective clinical decision making – like all competencies, you can practise and develop these alongside the acquisition of experience. The CHOICES mnemonic highlights some of these:

- **C**ritical thinking: involves remaining professionally curious, evaluating information from an objective perspective, avoiding emotion, recognising the risk of bias and challenging assumption.

- **H**euristics: recognising patterns, learning from experience and applying that learning to different circumstances.

- **O**thers: recognising sources of information, seeking advice from colleagues and the wider multidisciplinary team, sharing ideas and concerns.

- **I**ndividual reflection: reviewing decisions following the outcome, identifying missed opportunities to have made a different decision, and adjusting the future approach.

- **C**ommunication skills: proactively seeking information from both the patient and others involved in their care, active listening, recognising non-verbal cues and sharing information in an accessible way.

- **E**vidence base: familiarity with clinical practice guidelines and other sources of information to guide decisions, seeking clarification and confirmation where required rather than relying on memory.

- **S**hared approach: ensuring the patient remains fully involved in the decision-making process through the principle of 'no decision about me without me', sharing decisions with colleagues.

The importance of shared decision making is now well established within paramedic practice, but is still viewed with scepticism by many who consider it to be a threat to individual autonomy or a lack of trust by the employer. Many organisations mandate the use of shared decision making for NQPs which can add to the perception that it is linked to inexperience or inability. Despite this, involving others in critical or high-risk decisions invariably leads to reduced risk of error and better patient care. Within maternity services, a 'fresh eyes' approach to interpreting clinical findings not only reduced the risk of errors but also allowed midwives to support each other, presenting a learning process essential for professional practice (Donnelly and Hamilton, 2012). You may find that the act of preparing information for a remote clinical consultation with a colleague can be sufficient to identify gaps in your decision-making process, and for this reason shared decision making should always be viewed as a patient safety and individual learning tool rather than a hindrance.

💬 ADVICE

'I was always sceptical about shared decision making, until one day I was preparing to discharge a patient who had been challenging to assess. As I attempted to summarise the findings of a protracted assessment to my clinical supervisor, I realised that their presenting symptoms, with the irrelevant information removed, clearly warranted hospital transport. Since then, I have always been grateful for the requirement to share a discharge decision.'

1. Evidence	2. Reasoning	3. Implementation
• Clinical situation (acute and chronic) • Clinical practice guidelines • Patient values and wishes	• Identify options and contingencies • Balance patient benefits vs burdens • Recommend treatment	• Deliver safe treatment and/or transport • Communication (patient and healthcare providers) • Review and reflect

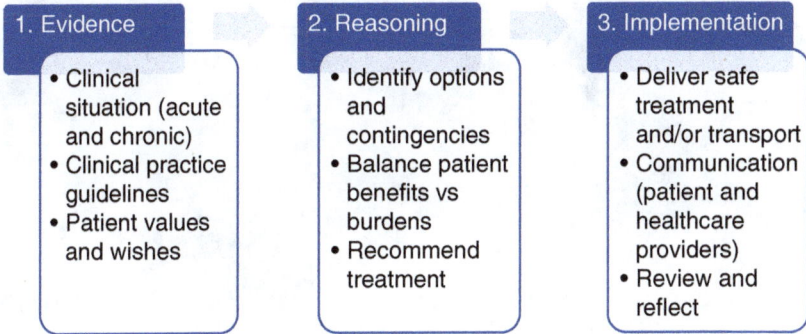

Figure 4.3 – Modified Warwick Model.

The Decision-making Process

There is no single correct way to make a decision, and a wide range of cognitive models exist to support clinicians. In simple terms, a decision rests between the input of information and the output of action, and this has been captured well within the Warwick Model (Bassford et al., 2019), which has been adapted for use by NQPs in clinical practice (Figure 4.3).

Chapter 5
Continuing Professional Development

Dr William Halsted, widely considered one of the founders of modern medicine, experimented with cocaine as an anaesthetic during the 1880s, and in doing so became addicted himself. Despite recognising the adverse impact on his health and career, Halsted later trialled the use of morphine to treat his cocaine addiction, consequently developing a morphine addiction which persisted for the remainder of his life (Wright and Schachar, 2020). Despite his significant contribution to the development of his profession, Halsted seemingly struggled with applying learning from his experiences, at least in this area of his practice.

What is Continuing Professional Development?

Put simply, continuing professional development (CPD) is any activity which leads to development of your skills, knowledge or ability. This can include formal activities such as completing accredited training courses, writing a reflective review of an individual experience, or undertaking eLearning – but there are many informal activities which can support professional development and are not as structured.

Almost a century ago, American philosopher and psychologist John Dewey identified that rather than learning from experience, we actually learn from reflecting on that experience (Dewey, 1933). Experience may lead to repetition and habit, but reflection allows us to apply meaning which can bring about growth or change. In real terms, it is reflection which allows us to adapt our behaviours and apply the effect of a decision (which may only be known after the decision is made) to similar future decisions.

Importance of Reflection

Reflective practice is the hallmark of an effective and professional practitioner, requiring you to critique your own strengths and weaknesses and take appropriate steps to improve your patient care. This is particularly relevant for NQPs, who are more likely to encounter novel or unfamiliar situations, and for whom a rapidly developing bank of experiences means that even common patient presentations are likely to offer unique perspectives. Circumstances which may have been familiar as a student paramedic can seem different when faced as a qualified and autonomous clinician, and although this can be a source of anxiety it can also present the best opportunities for professional growth. Vygotsky (1978) discusses the 'zone of proximal development' (ZPD), which he describes as a middling ground between what an individual is already capable of and what cannot be done by the same individual even with assistance (Figure 5.1). In clinical practice, this could be considered the area of practice which is currently slightly beyond your capabilities, but may be achievable with support.

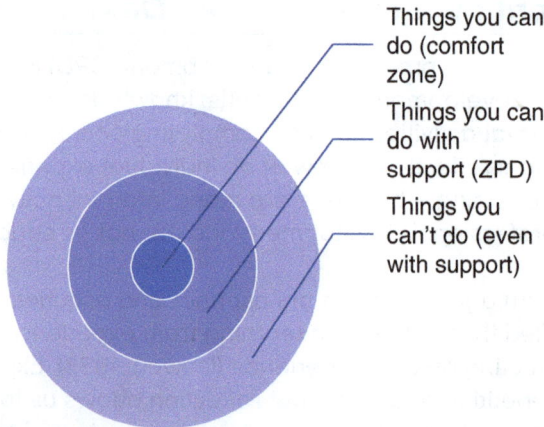

Things you can do (comfort zone)

Things you can do with support (ZPD)

Things you can't do (even with support)

Figure 5.1 – Zone of proximal development.

An example of this could relate to appropriate referral pathways. Immediately after starting, you may be aware of the need to refer certain patient groups, but not what referral pathways are available and therefore will require support with identifying these. On the next occasion, you may recall the available pathways but be unfamiliar with the acceptance criteria for each. As clinical competence and confidence increase, so too will the ability to refer in most cases without support. There will probably still be complex cases which push you outside of your comfort zone, but each presents an opportunity to learn for future similar presentations.

There are two key factors which will promote effective development in these situations: support and reflection (Phillips, 2024). Support may be co-located or remote, but is often dependent on your willingness to seek assistance, which in turn may be influenced by the perceived availability of that guidance. An organisational culture which supports learning will usually have mechanisms in place for this. By definition, tasks which sit within the zone of proximal development require support to achieve, to allow for future independence – in circumstances where you don't feel confident to act, you should always feel confident to ask.

Equally important is reflection, which gives you the opportunity to consider your actions and decisions more slowly, without having to be concerned about the impact of those decisions. By the time you reflect, the outcome (regardless of what it is) has usually occurred, and reflection therefore provides the opportunity to consider whether the outcome was appropriate or could have been improved in any way. A common misconception amongst NQPs is that 'reflection' refers to a formal activity, which must be written, often has a minimum word count, and will probably be reviewed by somebody else. In practice, reflecting on an action or decision can be nothing more than recognising that a decision wasn't effective and considering an alternative if faced with a similar situation again, and while it can be helpful to engage others in this very personal review of your actions, it is by no means a requirement.

> ### ✍ ACTIVITY
>
> Five-minute thoughts. If you struggle to get started with reflection, set a five-minute timer and commit to writing down, without structure, everything that comes to mind during this time. Continue without stopping or censoring yourself until the timer sounds. Be open and honest – nobody else needs to read it, but it can form the basis for a future reflective activity.

It is important to note that while every situation can lead to learning, not everything is an ideal learning opportunity. The further you move from your comfort zone, the more task focused you are likely to become and the less able to develop. It is essential that NQPs are supported to progress, and this is rarely achieved when attempting to complete seemingly impossible tasks. It is incumbent on employers to ensure a supportive working environment, and this should be a key factor for you when choosing where to work. Finding the balance to maximise opportunities to work within the zone of proximal development can be hard, but growth can be found between comfort and chaos.

Developing as a Reflective Practitioner

You will probably have developed your ability to reflect throughout your student paramedic programme, but this is often associated with a negative trigger – either prompted in practice by an event which has not gone as planned or required by a university assessment process (where the content may be guided). A key aspect of professional development is learning to reflect honestly, unencumbered by concerns around reputation or judgement for perceived mistakes. This requires reflection to take place within a 'safe space' which focuses on learning – ideally within an organisation which embeds a just culture.

There are many different theories and models which can help to guide you with reflection, but none are designed to be followed exclusively and the likelihood is that most practitioners will move between different models depending on the circumstances. Although reflection does not need to be a formal process, it does need to be an active one and requires a combination of the correct disposition and skill to achieve. Reflection is a skill which can be practised and enhanced, but requires a degree of underlying curiosity, discomfort and vulnerability to be most effective; this can be particularly challenging if you are already experiencing the negative effects of these emotions through a lack of confidence. Following a reflective model can provide an enforced structure which, rather than being restrictive (as often perceived), provides a permissive approach to analysing feelings and using these to develop. As you become more experienced, reflection is likely to evolve into an integrated part of your practice rather than a deliberate and separate activity.

✎ ACTIVITY

Are you a reflective practitioner? Reflection is a skill that can be developed but some people are naturally more reflective than others. Often this is associated with negative characteristics such as over-thinking or self-doubt, but by making reflection an intentional act with the motivation to improve practice, it can improve both confidence and competence. Use of a self-assessment tool such as the quiz provided by Lawrence-Wilkes and Ashmore (2014) can help with this.

Reflective Models

Reflective models vary in complexity and are often designed to be cyclical in nature, highlighting the importance of ongoing development and the application of learning to future situations. The simplest essence of reflection is best captured by Rolfe et al. (2001) which involves identifying the event, the meaning and any change required:

- **What** *happened*?
- **So what** does this *mean*?
- **Now what** do you need to *do*?

There are many different tools to choose from, and both personal preference and the purpose of the reflection can help determine the most appropriate tool to use, if any. Below are a selection of tools which are less commonly used within student paramedic programmes, but which are very applicable to practice as an NQP.

Greenaway et al. (2015) provide a slightly expanded approach with the Active Reviewing Cycle, which specifically incorporates feelings to encourage a deeper engagement with the impact of the event on you, in order to promote critical thinking:

- *Facts*: an objective account of the situation.
- *Feelings*: an honest report of your emotional response.
- *Findings*: a judgement of the learning you can take from the situation.
- *Future*: how you will apply this learning to other similar occurrences.

Some NQPs prefer to use a mnemonic approach to guide their reflective practice. The following model from Lawrence-Wilkes and Ashmore (2014) uses the word REFLECT as a prompt:

- **R**emember: recall an experience which you would like to change.
- **E**xperience: what happened and why is it significant in your memory?
- **F**ocus: consider any specific relevant details which may have affected the event.
- **L**earn: what went well, and less well. Why?
- **E**valuate: consider the effect of this experience on you, both good and bad.
- **C**onsider: what needs to change and how can you develop?
- **T**rial: create a specific action plan to implement the change you identified.

Finally, the College of Paramedics (2022a) has developed a reflective tool called WRAPT which has a particular focus on the well-being and emotional resilience of the practitioner, identifying the risks of upsetting or traumatic incidents and emphasising the importance of resilience and support. The WRAPT tool is available to access from the College of Paramedics website where you can create an online account to record your reflections.

- **W**ork: what are the details of the incident attended?
- **R**isks: what are the emotional risks as a result of attending this incident? Consider potential triggers outside work.
- **A**wareness: how did you feel at the time, and up to 72 hours afterwards? Are you aware of where you can access support?
- **P**lay: what are you going to do now to relax? How will you prepare yourself for the next shift?
- **T**hink: who can you share your reflection, thoughts or feelings with to improve your emotional well-being?

Peer Reflection

Although reflection is generally considered an individual activity, there is also merit in reflecting in a group setting, referred to as peer reflection. While the prospect of critically analysing your ability in front of others may feel daunting (particularly when discussing any perceived deficits), it is likely that you will have naturally instigated informal conversations with your peers, for example an informal debrief with your crewmate following an incident, sharing of experiences with other NQPs who have started at a similar time or a crew room conversation about a clinical hot topic. Aside from the benefits to CPD, this also supports emotional resilience through a shared understanding of the pressures of the workplace – a 'community of coping' (Korczynski, 2003). The greatest benefit of peer reflection is the opportunity to consider alternative perspectives that may be overlooked individually and capitalise on collective experience – the learning may be personal but 'no one knows as much as all of us' (McNicoll, 2008).

When participating in peer reflection, it is important that it remains mutually beneficial for all parties involved. While it can be an effective way to ameliorate concerns with performance, it can be equally effective to focus on what went well by highlighting good practice and the thought process which led to effective clinical decision making. An open questioning technique is key to these discussions – the TED acronym helps to ensure that questions remain open.

- **T**ell me...
- **E**xplain...
- **D**escribe...

> ### ✎ ACTIVITY
>
> Shared reflection. Within your workplace, arrange to meet regularly with a small group of colleagues, taking turns to present a case study and then discuss it as a group. Case studies can be fictitious or based on incidents attended, and don't forget to also reflect on what factors affected the promotion of efficacy.

Meeting Regulator Standards

As a regulated professional, you are required to adhere to the standards set by the regulator – the HCPC. The *Standards of Proficiency for Paramedics* (HCPC, 2023b) state that 'at the point of registration, paramedics must be able to... keep their skills and knowledge up to date and understand the importance of continuing professional development throughout their career'. This allows all registrants to practise safely throughout their career, and ensures that the public are protected from indoctrinated practice which often lacks any evidence base.

Verification of CPD is undertaken in two ways – the first is the biennial renewal cycle. All paramedics are required to re-register with the HCPC every two years (every other 1st of September), and at this stage you must complete a professional declaration that you have continued to practise (or met the requirements for returning to practice) and have met the standards for CPD. This is then audited through a random selection of 2.5% of paramedics being requested to submit a CPD profile to the HCPC for review, to demonstrate (with supporting evidence) how your CPD activities meet the standards. Although this is often a source of anxiety for paramedics, the process is not punitive and the vast majority of paramedics will have undertaken more CPD activity than is required. The hardest part is often ensuring this activity is recorded accurately and adequately, and developing good habits as an NQP by keeping a portfolio of development is recommended. NQPs enrolled in a preceptorship programme will usually be supported to maintain a portfolio of evidence as part of this, which will meet the standards expected by the HCPC – and continuing this portfolio following completion of preceptorship is likely to be the easiest way to continue meeting the standards. It is also worth noting that you will not be audited within your first two years of registration (HCPC, 2017), but following this will be subject to the same random selection approach.

ACTIVITY

Creating a CPD portfolio. There are numerous options for how you can effectively document the CPD you have undertaken, ranging from a paper-based ring binder of documents to online interactive ePortfolios. While individuals will often continue with a method they have been recommended to use during their student paramedic programme or provided by their employer, it is worth exploring the different systems available. Take the time to research some of the more popular portfolio options and decide which offers the most benefits for you – ideally one which will encourage frequent use!

During the audit process, the HCPC is ensuring that you meet its five CPD standards (HCPC, 2017). These are that registrants must:

1. Maintain a continuous, up-to-date and accurate record of CPD activities

2. Demonstrate that CPD activities are a mixture of learning activities relevant to current or future practice

3. Seek to ensure that CPD has contributed to the quality of their practice and service delivery

4. Seek to ensure that CPD benefits the service user

5. Upon request, present a written profile (which must be their own work and supported by evidence) explaining how they have met the standards for CPD.

💬 **ADVICE**

'I try to link my CPD with tasks I have to do anyway – when my employer sends out a clinical update I have to read, I'll record what I have learned.'

Making It Count – How to Ensure CPD Meets the Standards

To ensure that CPD activity meets the standards, you can follow the five Rs (Figure 5.2).

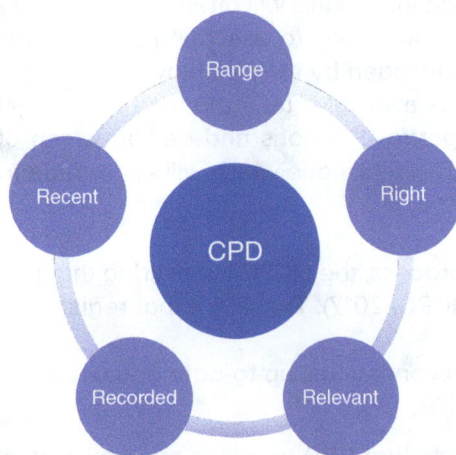

Figure 5.2 – The five Rs.

Range

Activities should cover a broad range of topics and a wide variety of methods. While you may feel most enthusiastic about exploring the area of specialism you intend to adopt which will inevitably (and appropriately) lead to a focus on learning to support this, CPD should cover the full spectrum of practice. Often it is the subjects which interest you the least where there is the most learning to be gained. Consider linking activities to the four pathways within the College of Paramedics (2024b) Career Framework.

> **💬 ADVICE**
>
> 'Little and often works for me. I try to make use of unexpected moments of free time, for example five minutes waiting for my crewmate to return, to learn something new and make a note on my phone.'

Right

Activities should be appropriate for your role and experience, and utilise a reliable source of information. It is important to differentiate between fact and opinion – both have their place but you must critically evaluate sources with regard to accuracy. When presenting written information, sources should be referenced appropriately to avoid plagiarism.

There are various standard formats for referencing which allow for uniformity in structure but there is no universally accepted format, meaning you can use your preferred method (including freeform) in your portfolio, as long as the source is identifiable.

Relevant

All learning should be relevant to your practice, meaning that it develops the quality of your practice and improves patient care. CPD activity might be aimed at supporting current development, but could also be intended to prepare you for a different role in the future as part of your career progression.

If you practise in an atypical or specialised work environment, it is appropriate for CPD activity to demonstrate how your role supports the delivery of clinical care within that environment, although it may also be useful to consider the wider aspects of the *Standards of Proficiency for Paramedics*.

> 💬 **ADVICE**
>
> 'Always link what you do back to the patient, after all, that's why we're all here in the first place.'

Recent

Evidence should be current – generally anything older than 24 months should be considered 'historical' and filed separately. While there are some exceptions to this (such as formal qualifications which have a specified validity period), the key word is 'continuous' – CPD should demonstrate ongoing and current activity.

Qualifications which are significant but no longer current can still be recorded within a curriculum vitae (CV) and can support future job applications or access to further learning, but generally a CV would not form a part of your CPD record.

Recorded

Continuing professional development undertaken should be evidenced and auditable – this is good practice for maintaining consistency in development, evaluating progress, supporting career progression and meeting regulator requirements. While CPD is a personal endeavour and there is generally no requirement to provide copies of any CPD activity to an employer, it can be helpful when evidencing progress against performance objectives, as part of an annual appraisal or for demonstrating career aspirations.

While anecdotally most paramedics undertake a vast range of both informal and formal CPD activity, there is little research evidencing the engagement of paramedics with CPD (Handyside and Watson, 2023) and the collective anxiety around being selected for CPD audit suggests that maintaining an accurate record of the activity undertaken remains a cause for concern.

> 💬 **ADVICE**
>
> 'Record it when you do it – if you wait until a later stage when you 'have time' it will get forgotten.'

Chapter 6
Clinical Leadership

Peter Drucker, who has been described as 'the founder of modern management' (Denning, 2014), wrote in his 1992 book *Managing for the Future* that 'a leader is someone who has followers' (Drucker, 1992). While this almost banal definition may seem simplistic, the point he is making is nonetheless significant: it doesn't matter how much experience you have, what your rank or seniority is or what leadership theory you choose to apply – unless you are able to motivate people to follow you, you're not a leader.

The importance of leadership in clinical practice is widely acknowledged but also widely defined. Leadership can be as specific as your individual actions as a clinician supporting others while providing direct patient care, and as broad as the executive-level oversight that senior management teams use to support an entire workforce. Despite the variance in definitions, leadership invariably involves behaviours or actions which are used to motivate individuals towards a common goal or a shared purpose, and within the clinical setting this shared purpose is generally the provision of high-quality patient care. This can be demonstrated formally, for example by taking on the 'team leader' role in a structured, high-acuity patient care episode such as managing a cardiac arrest, but can equally be observed informally in the way a clinician responds to feedback, communicates with peers and supports others. Informal leaders are often identified rather than appointed, and most clinical teams can usually identify who these leaders are – the people who others naturally gravitate towards for help and support.

For NQPs, the requirement to act as a clinical leader coincides with several other new expectations which can threaten to overload bandwidth and confidence. Particularly in the very early stages, when new experiences are at their peak, there is an understandable focus on individual actions and obligations, and the prospect of taking on responsibility for the actions, development and wellbeing of others is daunting; however, leadership is an expectation for the paramedic from the point of registration (HCPC, 2023b). Fortunately, 'newly qualified' and 'leader' can be symbiotic rather than opposing roles.

Leading a Scene

Understanding the specific circumstances where leadership is required can offer you a good starting point when wishing to develop your skills, with the initial focus commonly being on clinical leadership at the point of care. Following an initial period of direct support, you will often be the lead clinician on scene, expected not only to manage the patient correctly but also to provide direction and guidance to other colleagues present.

Leading a scene requires a combination of science (knowledge and understanding of the relevant evidence bases) and art (the field craft of choreographing the actions of others) which takes time to master, but once perfected can significantly reduce cognitive overload. The challenge is that every situation is different – a unique mix of the physical location, the people involved (both patients and clinicians) and their individual emotions and interactions. Add to this that scenes are rarely static, evolving in demand and complexity, and it's little wonder that scene leadership is a frequently cited source of concern. There is no magic recipe for resolving this, but applying the following principles may help to ease the pressure.

Control What Can Be Controlled

Maintaining control will reduce the number of unexpected events at the scene, making it easier to manage. Some environments are inherently more chaotic than others, but even where the choice of environment cannot be controlled, the way in which it is navigated can be – considerations such as moving the patient to a more private location or encouraging extraneous bystanders to move on can have a rapid positive impact. There is a limit to the number of spans of control that you can manage simultaneously, but reducing these where possible through the use of guidelines and checklists allows you to focus on the elements which require active decision making.

Delegate What Can Be Delegated

A common error made by inexperienced leaders is to try to do everything themselves, often believing this is easier than asking others to undertake the required task, or that there is a professional risk associated with delegation. As long as you delegate tasks to appropriate individuals, and employ closed loop communication both at the start ('Are you confident to...?') and end ('Let me know when you have...') of the task, the risk is minimal – and the cognitive bandwidth which can be freed by not performing a task is generally sufficient to monitor its progress.

Defer What Cannot Be Completed

Where an action cannot be completed for any reason (for example, insufficient resources, skillset or time), you will need to determine how essential that action is and then either take active steps to resolve the deficiency which is preventing it occurring or defer the action until a later point. Either way, there is little benefit in focusing on unachievable actions.

Ask for Help When Needed

Inexperienced leaders may worry that seeking help reduces credibility, but a key element of leadership is recognising your limitations. Asking for the appropriate help to manage a scene not only supports safe patient care but can also help provide a mitigation for the stress you may experience and allow you to manage the scene more effectively until that help arrives.

It's Not Over Until It's Over

A key element of leadership is caring for the team, including providing support following the conclusion of a patient care episode. While the benefits of undertaking a formal 'hot' debrief are debated, with poorly conducted debriefs risking ongoing psychological harm (Snowdon, 2021), it is still incumbent upon you to ensure that those for whom you are directly or vicariously responsible are safeguarded prior to dispersing. A simple but effective way of achieving this is using the TIPS mnemonic to review with the care team prior to closing the case:

- **T**hank you and well done: ensure team contribution is recognised.

- **I**mmediate risks: consider if there is anything requiring urgent escalation.

- **P**riority learning: focusing on improvement, not circumstantial learning needs.

- **S**afeguarding: are all team members safe to depart with appropriate support structures in place?

> ### 💬 ADVICE
>
> 'Talk through all your decisions out loud – this ensures the whole team knows what you are planning (and why), but also gives you an automatic safety check.'

Clinical Leadership

In a broader sense, acting as a clinical leader involves demonstrating, and encouraging others to demonstrate, the knowledge, skills and attributes which result in high-quality patient care. Despite the tight focus of an individual patient encounter, interactions rarely take place in isolation and all patient care is a product of the system within which it occurs. Therefore, while it can be tempting to take a narrow view, focusing your efforts on your individual actions, all practitioners need to maintain awareness of the impact of those actions on others. The Butterfly Effect has become well known in popular culture (the concept that a butterfly flapping its wings in one continent can influence the path of a tornado in another), but this same principle can apply to most clinical decisions regardless of the clinical setting: all actions have consequences. Adverse outcomes do not make a decision fundamentally poor, but it is essential to remain cognisant of the potential unintended impacts. NQPs often proudly discuss their autonomy but with great autonomy comes great responsibility – and clinical leadership requires that responsibility to be wielded wisely.

💬 **ADVICE**

'Sounding confident when instructing others is essential – if you don't, no matter how correct you are, there will always be a degree of uncertainty in those you are directing.'

Many of the skills which you will develop are transferrable to both on-scene and wider clinical leadership. These relate to clinical ability, problem solving, communication, decision making and risk assessment. When combined with a sound underpinning of clinical knowledge, these skills can allow you to develop a strong leadership ability from the outset. However, to truly develop clinical leadership, there are several attributes which it is necessary to refine. Cook and Leathard (2004) highlight five:

1. *Creativity*: actively engaging to seek novel approaches.

2. *Highlighting*: promoting new ideas and challenging inertia.

3. *Influencing*: using information to inspire others.

4. *Respecting*: recognising and responding to non-verbal indicators.

5. *Supporting*: guiding, rather than directing, others.

Irrespective of your stage of career development, you should be seeking opportunities to demonstrate these attributes within your work. At the most fundamental level, they form the basis for sound clinical leadership, but if you aspire to future leadership or managerial positions then adopting these attributes as a basis allows them to become second nature throughout your career journey.

ACTIVITY

How could you apply the five attributes of clinical leadership when supervising other clinicians within your working environment? What challenges might you face?

Followership

If a leader is someone who has followers, then it stands to reason that followership is an equally important skill – in fact, part of being a clinical leader is about recognising when to follow. Despite how it sounds, the role of the follower is not passive, undertaking several important functions within a team:

- Support the leader's decision making
- Perform delegated tasks confidently and effectively
- Contribute ideas and suggestions
- Hold the leader accountable and challenge where necessary.

The latter responsibility is easily overlooked, but particularly for NQPs who may be required to move seamlessly (and repeatedly) between the leader and follower role, it is important to be aware that your accountability does not cease when there is another leader involved.

ACTIVITY

The reasons why people choose to follow a leader range from negative (mandated, lack of better options) to positive (logical agreement, shared vision). When leading, how can you motivate your team to follow you for the right reasons?

Leadership Theories and Strategies

Despite an ever-increasing volume of published research relating to the subject, and a ubiquitous acceptance of the importance of leadership skills within healthcare, a universally accepted definition of leadership remains elusive, and theories are often variable in terms of their acceptance and application. In reality, it is often easier to recognise a good leader than it is to identify what makes them effective, and maintaining an awareness of some of the more well-known theories can help you to develop your own leadership style.

For much of the 20th century, research focused on individuals and the prevailing view was that leaders were born, not made. Often referred to as trait theory, research focused on identifying the innate characteristics which made a great leader – and a large number of traits were identified. The challenge was that the correlation between these traits and 'great leadership' was minimal and inconsistent (Mann, 1959).

By focusing on these individual traits, Lewin et al. (1939) identified three distinct leadership styles:

- *Autocratic*: makes decisions independently and directs others.

- *Laissez-faire*: leaves others to make decisions and remains uninvolved.

- *Democratic*: encourages everybody to contribute before making final decision.

Although democratic leadership is highlighted as the preferred style, certain circumstances may require other forms of leadership. The ability to move between styles as dictated by the situation is important, which suggests leadership ability is not a fixed trait but situation dependent.

Situational leadership follows the premise that there is no single best approach to leadership, and that the method used should vary based on two factors: the task and the people (or relationships) involved

(Hersey and Blanchard, 1969). For NQPs, working in unpredictable environments with changing teams, the four leadership behaviours of situational leadership are all likely to be desirable at different times:

- *Delegating* (low task behaviour, low relationship behaviour): leaders monitor progress but delegate decisions to the group.

- *Participating/supporting* (low task behaviour, high relationship behaviour): leaders focus on relationships to work with the team and encourage shared decisions.

- *Coaching* (high task behaviour, high relationship behaviour): leaders provide the direction but coach others to deliver this.

- *Telling/directing* (high task behaviour, low relationship behaviour): leaders provide clear commands.

Following widespread acceptance of situational theory, adaptations and enhancements led to a new paradigm of approaches, the best known of which is Burns' (1978) Transformational Leadership Theory. This style of leadership focuses on inspiring and motivating followers to work towards a set of shared objectives, with leaders 'transforming' people to help them perform at their best. While the antithesis, 'transactional leadership', assumes that followers are motivated by what they receive in return for their followership (in the workplace this might be performance in exchange for their salary, but from a clinical perspective this could be perceived as individual actions motivated by a positive outcome), transformational leadership is about developing individuals to perform at their best, regardless of specific outcomes.

Notwithstanding your individual preferences or future career aspirations, an adaptable leadership style which acknowledges the unique requirements of the situation and the team, and prioritises developing the capability of others, is likely to be most effective in both clinical practice and wider professional interactions. NHS England (2023b) recognises the importance of leadership amongst paramedics, and highlights the dimensions that should be developed at both foundational and developmental career stages. Utilising the support of your preceptorship to develop this foundation provides a strong basis for future clinical and leadership roles.

Human Factors and Crew Resource Management

On the 29th of March 2005, Elaine Bromiley attended hospital for an elective routine operation. Less than an hour later, she had suffered irreversible brain damage from which she sadly died 13 days later. Her death was not the result of any underlying condition or illness, but due to a cascade of errors in judgement made by the clinicians responsible for her safety. None of these clinicians were incompetent, poorly trained or wishing to cause harm – they simply made human decisions in circumstances that required a more structured, systematic approach (Clinical Human Factors Group, 2005).

The human element of patient care is, for the most part, one of the biggest influences on patient experience – without humanity, there can be no compassion or empathy. When recalling experiences of receiving healthcare, it is overwhelmingly the behaviours of the healthcare staff that patients remember, far beyond any clinical assessment or treatment which may have taken place. But sometimes these human qualities which lead to great patient care can also be the cause of iatrogenic harm. The study of human factors in healthcare aims to recognise, and therefore minimise, this risk.

Recognising human factors has its roots in aviation, where NASA research in the 1970s identified that contrary to popular belief at the time, the majority of aircraft accidents were not caused by mechanical breakdown but by the inability of crews to respond adequately to an unexpected situation (Cooper et al., 1979). The incorporation of Crew Resource Management (CRM) training to support human interaction with complex systems using communication tools, decision-making support, workload distribution and error identification has resulted in the airline industry leading the way in safety. Conversely, medicine has been slow to adopt these principles, despite a seminal report from the Institute of Medicine (2000), *To Err is Human*, highlighting an epidemic of patient harm which is often illustrated as more people dying through medical error than if a jumbo jet were to crash every day.

For the NQP, this is a sobering and alarming fact. The perceived professional and ethical consequences of making any mistake are significant, let alone one which results in patient death – and as an inexperienced practitioner this risk feels more likely. However, this concern can also act as an effective safeguard to mitigate the risk, through a heightened awareness of the human factors which are likely to lead to error if not considered. This is not a single panacea to prevent harm, as Reason's (1997) Swiss Cheese Model highlights that fallibility exists through multiple human and systems errors aligning, but it does help you to develop your clinical practice in a way which minimises risk.

There is no comprehensive list of precursors to human error, since every situation is unique, but DuPont (1997) summarised the 12 most common causes for aircraft maintenance personnel to make errors in judgement, and this so-called 'dirty dozen' (Table 6.1) has been widely considered in all fields of work due to its relevance. The remainder of this section will focus on these, grouped into similar themes to create a 'filthy five'. As you will often be the clinical lead on scene, these factors should be recognised and mitigated for the entire care team.

Table 6.1 – The human factors 'dirty dozen'.

Presence of:		Inadequate:	
1	Distraction	7	Communication
2	Stress	8	Resources
3	Complacency	9	Teamwork
4	Pressure	10	Awareness
5	Fatigue	11	Knowledge
6	Norms	12	Assertiveness

ACTIVITY

For each of the case studies presented below, reflect on whether you have experienced a similar situation and how you could adjust your practice to minimise the risk.

Distraction and Lack of Awareness

Sources of distraction can be either intrinsic or extrinsic. Inexperience can increase the risk of distraction due to a reduced ability to filter extraneous information sources, and therefore self-regulation to focus on what is most relevant is essential. Distraction can also lead to a reduction in situational awareness and a focus on the details rather than the bigger picture. In general activity, the human mind works much quicker than the hands and so thinking ahead is common; however, any distraction risks physical tasks being missed as your mind is already thinking about starting the next assignment rather than completing the current one.

Countermeasures include:

- Avoiding the temptation to multi-task, which is rarely effective (try humming one song while listening to another)
- Utilising checklists where available (the algorithms in JRCALC are ideal for this)
- Using visual reminders for outstanding tasks
- Utilising automated audible prompts (for example, setting an alarm which sounds every five minutes)
- Physically stepping backwards to maintain a wider field of vision
- Challenging thought processes with 'what if' scenarios.

Case study

Strokes are time-critical emergencies, with very few prehospital interventions required, but a recent study found average on-scene times in excess of 30 minutes (McClelland et al., 2023). This is unlikely to be due to a lack of awareness of the need for rapid transport, but due to distractions while on scene resulting in time 'running away'.

Inadequate Communication or Teamwork

Breakdown in communication is common, often due to a focus on the passive sending of information without confirming receipt. When communicating verbally, the message is more than simply what you say – consider how urgency is often inferred through tone of voice. Many childhood games demonstrate how easily communication can break down when passed via an intermediary, and the risk is increased in high-pressure circumstances. Poor communication inevitably influences teamwork, and regardless of who takes clinical lead, healthcare is a team effort with no single person solely responsible for safe and effective outcomes.

Countermeasures include:

● Utilising tools and mnemonics to share information (Table 6.2)

● Starting a message with the most important information, repeating at the end if necessary

● Ensuring all team members are appropriately briefed and understand their role

Table 6.2 – SBAR handover tool.

Situation	Introduce those involved, identify reason for the communication.
Background	Provide relevant context which will support decision making.
Assessment	Key influencing factors and options considered.
Recommendation	Suggested outcome with desired timeframe.

Source: based on NHS Institute for Innovation and Improvement, 2010.

- Using 'closed loop' communication by requesting (and giving) verbal confirmation when an action is completed

- Where appropriate, following up verbal directions with written confirmation.

Case study

Passing a hospital pre-alert is often considered stressful, particularly for inexperienced clinicians (Sampson et al., 2024). Following a consistent approach which focuses on essential information reduces cognitive load and increases clarity.

> 💬 **ADVICE**
>
> 'Speak to people by name (ask first if necessary) – not only does it prevent confusion about who's doing what, but it is just generally nicer.'

Stress, Pressure and Fatigue

Stress is a normal response to the pressure experienced when demands are placed upon an individual's senses. Acute stress happens in real time in response to an emerging 'threat' and supports the body's ability to deal with the situation through a physiological response – often recognised as the 'fight or flight' response. There are other manifestations to stress, however, which are more common but potentially less advantageous – specifically freezing (alongside 'flop' and 'friend') which occurs most frequently in inexperienced people (Vít et al., 2023).

Chronic stress accumulates over time, for example due to long-term illness, grief or workplace difficulties. This lowers the threshold for acute stress reactions and therefore can lead to rapid or extreme escalations in behaviour under moderate or even mild pressure.

Fatigue is the natural response to prolonged physical or mental stress, and can result from either the intensity or duration of the workload. This can be exacerbated through insufficient rest periods between work and the impact of fatigue is often insidious, with individuals perceiving that they can counteract the effects of fatigue rather than resolving the root cause or keeping concerns hidden due to fear of adverse consequences (Lombardo et al., 2024).

Countermeasures include:

- Addressing causes of long-term stress using health and well-being services both in and out of work, maintaining a healthy diet, remaining active and avoiding unhealthy habits

- Recognising the physical signs of stress in oneself and others, and seeking or offering support

- Utilising 'time out' when making critical decisions – breathe in and then out, slowly, and force yourself to delay the decision until this is completed

- Utilising shared decision making

- Reflecting on whether pressure is self-induced – being willing to delay non-urgent tasks (Table 6.3)

- Ensuring suitable and meaningful rest periods between hours of work.

Case study

There is little research exploring the resilience of NQPs (Phillips, 2024), but it is common for NQPs to undertake high amounts of overtime during the early stages of their career. Whether financially motivated, a novel enthusiasm for professional identity or born of a desire to expedite experience, this practice can result in insufficient rest, increased risk of error and premature onset of burnout.

Table 6.3 – The 4 Ds of time management.

	Not important	Important
Not urgent	Drop	Defer
Urgent	Delegate	Do

Source: adapted from the Eisenhower Matrix (Wise, 1991).

Inadequate Knowledge or Resources

A key attribute of paramedicine is the ability to provide a hospital standard of care in prehospital locations, with only the resources which can be carried in a vehicle and the knowledge of the attending clinicians. This can feel like a difficult challenge to overcome, particularly when you are working in rural or remote locations and the nearest clinical back-up may be some distance away. NQPs therefore become adept at adapting and making the most of what is available.

Other countermeasures include:

- Using guidelines to clarify information at the point of care, rather than relying on memory
- Ensuring equipment checks are completed correctly
- Escalating concerns with missing or unserviceable equipment
- Asking for back-up early (this can always be stood down if no longer required)
- Considering whether tasks (or parts of tasks) can be postponed until more resources are available – or whether the patient can be transported somewhere with appropriate resources
- Maintaining CPD.

Case study

The early stages of cardiac arrest management frequently stretch available resources and can be a defining moment for NQPs. Tuttle and Hubble (2018) found that paramedics who had been exposed to 15 or more resuscitations over five years were over 20% more likely to deliver a successful outcome.

Complacency, Norms and Lack of Assertiveness

Complacency could be considered the reverse of stress, where a lack of concern results in reduced awareness of potential risks. There is an increased likelihood of complacency during routine tasks which have become habitual, or during tasks which you consider 'safe'. This leads to an increased tendency to take chances, bypass steps (particularly safety elements which are included 'just in case' but which rarely result in findings) or rely on muscle memory rather than active decision making. This often manifests as normal behaviour, which becomes organisational culture. Bad habits embed far more easily than good ones, and culture can be described as 'the collection of behaviours which we tolerate'. Unfortunately, this can make it difficult to challenge poor practice (particularly when much of the time poor practice does not overtly lead to poor outcomes), and you may find it particularly difficult to challenge senior or more experienced colleagues.

Countermeasures:

- Remaining aware of conscious and unconscious bias, and the associated risks

- Always having a back-up plan (Table 6.4)

- Looking for anomalies, and seeking explanations for these

- Utilising a progressive escalation strategy for highlighting concerns (Table 6.5)

- Always being open to receiving professional challenges, particularly from junior colleagues.

Table 6.4 – Plan ABC.

Plan A	Aim	The primary goal to achieve the best outcome.
Plan B	Back-up	An alternative if plan A fails.
Plan C	Critical	A rapid and effective failsafe.

Table 6.5 – PACE tool for graded assertiveness.

Probe	'What is the correct route for adrenaline in anaphylaxis?'
Alert	'Are you going to administer intravenously?'
Challenge	'For anaphylaxis the adrenaline should be intramuscular'
Emergency	'Stop – you are about to make a medication error'

Source: based on Besco, 1995

Case study

Chest pain is commonly seen by paramedics but in younger age groups the cause is far more likely to be non-cardiac, which can lead to cognitive biases when forming a clinical impression (Gale, 2017) and adversely influence assessment and treatment decisions. This can be exacerbated where experienced colleagues are dismissive of the concerns of junior clinicians.

Chapter 7
Overcoming Challenges

In the 15th century, the Japanese military commander Ashikaga Yoshimasa returned a damaged tea bowl to China, where it had been made. The bowl was returned poorly repaired with ugly metal staples, prompting Japanese craftsmen to seek a more aesthetic means of restoration. The art of kintsugi was born, where damaged ceramics were bonded using a lacquer mixed with gold – the result often being so visually appealing that the repaired item was more valuable than it had been previously (Bartlett, 2008). Kintsugi stems from a Japanese philosophy that breakage and repair are part of the history of an object, to be celebrated rather than hidden – similarly for NQPs, challenges should be seen as overt opportunities for development rather than errors to be concealed.

When you first undertake independent clinical practice, you will inevitably find yourself in difficult and stressful situations but as experience increases, the number of novel occurrences is reduced and your bank of similar circumstances which can be used as a reference point increases, leading to a natural reduction in stress and improved degree of confidence. However, this change does not occur linearly, and can be affected by a range of intrinsic and extrinsic factors including:

- Breadth of exposure
- Actual and perceived support received
- Complexity of clinical cases attended
- Working environment
- Time away from clinical practice.

Although your individual experiences will vary, most NQPs go through broadly the same phases of development – an evolution in practice (Limmer, 2015) (Figure 7.1).

Just as tempering metal increases durability, repeatedly applying pressure to an NQP often increases resilience, but this can be dependent on how you react to, and are supported during, the 'reality check' moment. This chapter focuses on what this means, and how to overcome any challenges associated with the transition.

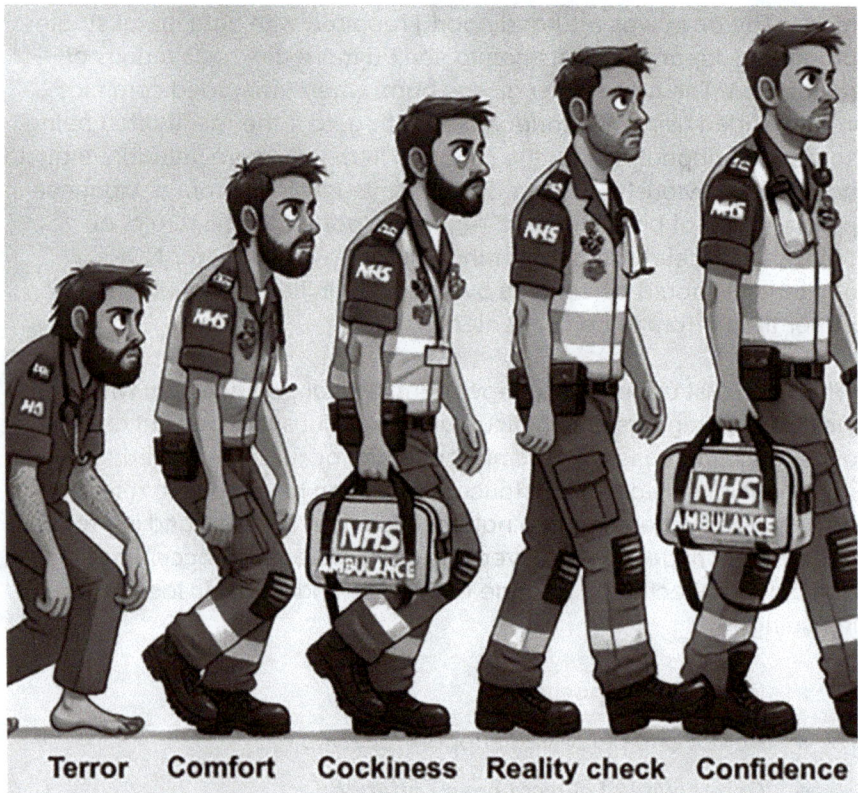

Terror   Comfort   Cockiness   Reality check   Confidence

Figure 7.1 – Evolution of practice.
Source: Adapted from Limmer (2015).

Accountability and Responsibility

Two words which are frequently used adjacently, sometimes misused interchangeably, but nonetheless have differing implications. This is further complicated by the fact that dictionaries often define one word in relation to the other (dictionary.com, 2025):

- *Responsibility*: 'answerable or accountable, as for something within one's power, control or management.'

- *Accountable*: 'subject to the obligation to report, explain, or justify something; responsible.'

The HCPC (2024) highlights that 'as a registrant, you are personally responsible for the way you behave'. This promotes the paramedic as an autonomous practitioner, able to make independent decisions but required to take ownership of those decisions and any resultant consequences. This does not mean mistakes cannot occur but does require you to accept those mistakes, be open and honest about them and take corrective action where possible. This may include making amends, apologising where appropriate and taking steps to learn from the error and minimise the likelihood of reoccurrence.

Accountability takes the premise of responsibility and adds the requirement to provide explanations for actions you have taken ownership for. This is often described as justifying any decisions which have been made, although the term 'justify' can sometimes imply an element of blame, and therefore a better description may be to explain the rationale for decisions and actions. A clear example of this lies in the completion of patient clinical records, where regardless of the form they take, best practice involves documenting what your patient assessment has revealed and how that has led to your chosen clinical management plan.

There is a further step beyond accountability, which is liability. This adds an element of external scrutiny where you may be judged for your actions, with reference to a formal framework, best practice or a consensus of peers. It is this which may cause you the most apprehension, particularly if you have low confidence or limited experience. Despite this concern, the hierarchy of responsibility (Figure 7.2) is an inevitable consequence of professional decision making and supports safe practice. Being aware of this, accepting that all your actions have consequences (some of which may be unforeseen) and remaining open to career-long learning allows professional responsibility to be seen as a positive aspect of your practice.

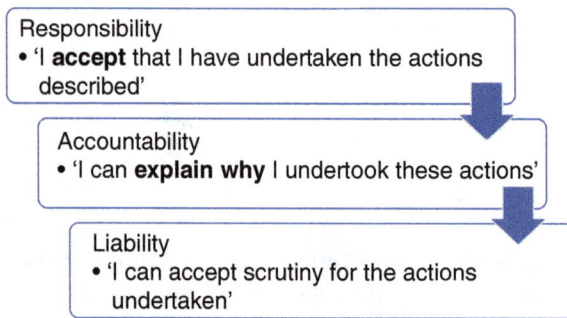

Responsibility
• 'I **accept** that I have undertaken the actions described'

Accountability
• 'I can **explain why** I undertook these actions'

Liability
• 'I can accept scrutiny for the actions undertaken'

Figure 7.2 – Hierarchy of responsibility.

✍ ACTIVITY

Think of an occasion when your actions had an unintended consequence which affected another person. How did you (or could you) act to demonstrate your responsibility and accountability for the situation? Were you held liable on this occasion?

Giving, Receiving and Learning from Feedback

Feedback is a critical component for growth. In much the same way as reflection allows you to critically analyse your actions, feedback provides insight into how those actions are perceived by others. This offers valuable understanding of performance, reinforces strengths and can highlight areas for development.

Newly qualified paramedics work within a dynamic team environment, resulting in diverse opportunities for sharing feedback. In the early stages of your career, you may prefer to focus on personal progression, seeking guidance and gaining reassurance on your practice. As confidence grows and you begin supervising junior grades, the ability to give feedback effectively gains significance. A common learning objective of preceptorship programmes is to develop mentoring skills which, while not usually expected of the NQP, are a key role of the experienced paramedic. Alongside clinical growth, therefore, the ability to support and develop others should also form part of your learning.

The purpose of feedback is generally to raise the recipient's awareness about their performance, with the intent of influencing their future decisions and actions. This is distinct from an immediate corrective action or instruction which may be needed to avoid harm, and therefore the way in which it is delivered should reflect this. Generally, feedback is either corrective or to reinforce good practice, and in both cases should be looking to future practice rather than the past – Goldsmith (2002) coined the term 'feedforward' to highlight this approach. As taught by the Dalai Lama (2019), and more recently by Rafiki in *The Lion King* (1994), we can't change the past, but we can learn from it – consequently, it is more constructive to help people be right than to prove they were wrong.

Most people already give feedback many times each day, often without realising and sometimes without intending to do so. Frequently this is brief and non-verbal, such as a smile in response to a kind word or a frown in response to an undesired offer. Conversely, few individuals perceive themselves as receiving regular feedback, which may be down to the way in which feedback is given or received, exacerbated by a failure to think forwards or focus on the intended impact of that feedback.

Principles of Effective Feedback

There are many published models which can be applied to support effective feedback in practice, summarised through the following key principles which help to ensure that whatever method is used, you can give, and receive, feedback effectively.

- *Timing*: most scholars suggest that feedback should be given as soon as possible following the event, to ensure it is fresh in the mind of both parties (Race, 2001). There are exceptions, though – giving feedback while still experiencing an emotional response to a situation (such as anger or anxiety) may result in a negative approach which fails to focus on improvement (Snowdon, 2021).

- *Trust*: maintain an environment of psychological safety, where those involved are allies with aligned goals. Where the recipient doubts the motivation of the person providing feedback, they are less likely to recognise or reflect on the information shared (Wiliam, 2011).

- *Truth*: giving feedback can be difficult, particularly if there is a fear it will be received negatively. Unfortunately, this can lead to generic comments which can be downplayed but are not effective or helpful. Try to ensure that all feedback is truthful and specific (Table 7.1).

- *Tact*: receiving feedback is equally difficult, and it is useful to recognise where an individual has already identified areas for development through reflection, as there is rarely any benefit in lengthy exploration of learning which is already known.

- *Thanks*: it is important to accept feedback with gratitude. As well as keeping the discourse positive (even if the feedback was not!), it prevents the feedback session becoming a debate, as any learning is likely to follow reflection rather than be immediate.

- *Two-way*: regardless of any disparity in qualifications or experience between individuals, it is rare for learning opportunities to be purely one-sided. Although the development need may vary, a feedback conversation will generally offer an opportunity for learning by all involved.

Table 7.1 – Examples of generalised versus specific feedback.

Area	Generic	Specific
Be specific	'Time management is poor'	'You appeared rushed to finish the patient assessment'
Take ownership	'Others have said that...'	'I have noticed that...'
Avoid evaluation	'Your physical examination was low standard'	'Your physical examination did not follow a structure'
Be factual	'You were too slow to...'	'It took you three minutes to...'
Actions, not personality	'You are too chatty'	'You interrupted the patient...'

ACTIVITY

Consider occasions when you have received feedback from someone, and list the factors which made it either a positive or negative experience. Next, think of when you have provided feedback, and consider which of these factors may have been perceived by the recipient. Reflect on how you can use this activity to influence any future feedback you provide.

Just Culture

Many organisations promote a learning culture, which is described by the CQC (2024) as 'a proactive and positive culture of safety based on openness and honesty, in which concerns about safety are listened to, safety events are investigated and reported thoroughly, and lessons are learned to continually identify and embed good practices'. Central to this is the assumption that people are not generally malicious, and therefore when harm occurs it is usually unintended, and often the consequence of a series of systemic failings which have permitted an individual error. For example, if an NQP discharges a patient from care inappropriately and that patient subsequently worsens, it may be the decision by the NQP which ultimately led to harm, but it was the system that permitted the patient to be discharged without further clinical oversight.

There are exceptions, however. High-profile cases such as that of Lucy Letby can undermine the aspiration to embed a learning culture, and underscore the importance of holding to account individuals who deliberately cause harm or are grossly negligent. A just culture requires an atmosphere of trust which encourages error reporting, but also clearly delineates where behaviours are unacceptable (Reason, 1997). Finding this balance can be challenging, as employee behaviours are driven by organisational culture. Culpability models can help guide decision making and differentiate between human error and deliberate violation, but human behaviour is nuanced and therefore every case or action must be considered in isolation.

The National Patient Safety Agency (NPSA) (2003) developed a decision tool to promote a consistent and fair approach in differentiating between individual causes and system failures. It utilises four sequential tests.

1. *Deliberate harm test*: were the actions, and any adverse consequences, intended?

2. *Incapacity test*: is there evidence of ill health or medical cause?

3. *Foresight test*: were there known and appropriate processes which the individual deviated from, or took an unacceptable risk?

4. *Substitution test*: would another similar individual in similar circumstances have acted similarly?

In practice, these tests can be used to guide your clinical decision making and minimise risk. By ensuring there is no intent to cause harm (consider the ubiquitous principle of medical ethics, first do no harm), that you remain fit to practise, that you are cognisant of and adhere to clinical practice guidelines and that your actions are consistent with those of other NQPs, then your decision is likely to be sound and, just as importantly, defensible.

In 2022, the Patient Safety Incident Response Framework (PSIRF) was published as a standardised approach for identifying learning from patient safety incidents, reinforcing a just and learning culture throughout the NHS. It focuses on a compassionate approach for those affected by, and involved in, patient safety incidents and seeks to deliver a considered and proportionate response which leads to systemic improvement.

The unpredictable nature of clinical practice means that you are likely to be involved in a patient safety incident investigation (PSII) at some point during your career, and this can be a daunting prospect. Alongside seeking support from peers or organisational leadership teams, it is important to understand that these investigations are not designed to attribute blame or hold individuals accountable, but instead to understand how an organisation's systems and processes contributed to the incident. Despite the anxiety caused, a PSII can be a beneficial learning activity which allows for reflection, insight and improved individual practice alongside organisational improvements.

Duty of Candour

When things do go wrong, one of the most important considerations is to be open and honest with those involved, including the patient. The Duty of Candour is both a statutory and professional obligation, and although the prompt for each varies, they are consistent in the requirement for an honest declaration, a meaningful apology and a commitment to understand what caused the adverse event, with a focus on preventing reoccurrence.

Professional (Ethical) Obligation

The professional duty applies directly to the individual clinician and arises from the HCPC (2024) *Standards of Conduct, Performance and Ethics*. Standard 8 requires you to 'be open when things go wrong'. In practice, this means that whenever an error is made, regardless of how minor, it is important that the patient is made aware. Ideally, this would be at the time of the error, with an explanation of the likely impact and the steps which are being taken to correct the mistake, and should also include an apology. Where it is not possible to exercise this duty contemporaneously, it may be necessary to seek support from your employer – and in all cases your employer's internal procedures should also be followed.

Statutory (Legal) Obligation

The legal duty is stipulated within Regulation 20 of the Health and Social Care Act 2008 (Regulated Activities) Regulations 2014 and applies to all organisations registered with the CQC. This responsibility sits with the organisation rather than the individual, and failure to comply can lead to criminal sanctions. Unlike the professional requirements, a legal duty only exists when there has been a notifiable safety incident; in other words, where an incident results in 'death... severe harm, moderate harm, or prolonged psychological harm' (CQC, 2022).

Practical Application

On a human level, being open about mistakes and apologising is a relatively common and straightforward occurrence. Within clinical practice, there are several factors which can make this more challenging:

- Fear of consequences
- Shared responsibility amongst the care team
- Prioritising ongoing life-saving treatment
- Mistakes are sometimes identified after the care episode has ended.

These factors may be exacerbated when the consequences of the error are more severe.

> ### ✎ ACTIVITY
>
> Consider the last time you were the victim of a mistake. Reflect on what happened, and what actions by the person who made the mistake could have, or did, make the situation better or worse. How could you apply this to your clinical practice?

When applying the Duty of Candour, consider the following.

1. Be genuine. It is rare for harm to have occurred deliberately. Be open about what has happened, and your apology will naturally be more candid.

2. Be prompt. Keeping the patient informed early often leads to a quicker, and more satisfactory, resolution.

3. Being open or apologising does not mean accepting legal liability – a regulator would view this as evidence of insight.

4. Document what happened, and the steps taken to rectify the situation (including any Duty of Candour discussions).

5. Seek support – both when communicating with the patient and for ongoing welfare support.

6. Learn. Anybody can make a mistake, and they rarely arise through malice or intent, but should be exploited to minimise the risk of repetition.

Fitness to Practise

All NQPs must have the required skills, knowledge, health and character to safely and effectively practise as a paramedic – collectively, this is referred to as 'fitness to practise'. Maintaining fitness to practise is your individual responsibility, and registered professionals are expected to take all necessary steps to do so. Assurance of fitness to practise is provided by the HCPC, which has a legislated mandate to investigate and, where necessary, take action to ensure that this is maintained in the UK paramedic workforce. Concerns can only be considered in relation to one of five statutory grounds: misconduct; lack of competence; conviction or caution; physical or mental health; or where there has been a determination by another regulatory body.

Where a paramedic's fitness to practise may be impaired, concerns can be raised with the HCPC through one of three routes – as a member of the public (including patients, relatives, colleagues or other agencies); as an employer; or by the registrant themselves. The latter, known as a self-referral, is significant, as where a paramedic self-refers it indicates that they have a degree of insight into any concerns about their practice. However, it is also an area of risk, as self-referrals by paramedics are disproportionately high and are often unwarranted (van der Gaag et al., 2017). Referrals should only be made where there is a genuine belief that professional standards have been breached, and concerns will generally be investigated and managed by the employer in the first instance. It is only where the employer has identified a substantial breach (or has found it necessary to restrict or suspend the paramedic's practice) that a referral should be made.

The fear of HCPC referral is significant amongst NQPs, exacerbated by HCPC registration being perceived as a subtle threat to encourage good practice – linguistically, terms such as 'protecting' registration or 'being struck off as a punishment' are common. While maintaining professional standards is undoubtedly important, the remit of the HCPC is not punitive and instead focuses on a single aim – to protect the public. To this end, fitness to practise sanctions are always forward facing – in other words, ensuring the public are safe from the registrant's future actions, regardless of what has happened in the past.

The Process

A fitness to practise process can take several years to reach an outcome, although many referrals are completed more quickly than this (particularly where there is found to be no case to answer). This is because there are several stages which need to be completed to ensure the process remains fair (Table 7.2).

Table 7.2 – Stages of fitness to practise process.

Stage	What's happening?
Triage	The concern is checked to ensure it relates to a current registrant, has been made in writing, and relates to one of the five statutory grounds.
Investigation	A case manager is assigned and fact-finding commences, to decide whether the concern meets the threshold to progress. If met, the concern will be formalised as one or more allegations, and these will be sent to the registrant with the opportunity to respond. The investigation details and registrant's response will be reviewed by a panel of three independent people (including a paramedic), who will determine if there is a case to answer.
Interim order	If there is a perceived risk to the public while proceedings take place, there may be an additional hearing to consider an interim order – this is a temporary restriction or suspension in practice until the final hearing is concluded.
Substantive (final) hearing	An adversarial tribunal hearing where the HCPC will formally present the allegations and associated evidence, and the registrant is given the opportunity to challenge them. An independent panel will then decide whether the allegations are well founded, and if so, whether the registrant's fitness to practise remains impaired. The panel may impose a sanction on the registrant if it is deemed necessary to protect the public or otherwise in the public interest.

Possible Sanctions

The sanctions which may be applied to a registrant following a final hearing are as follows:

- *Mediation*: intended to resolve minor issues by facilitating discussion to reach a mutual understanding between the registrant and another party.

- *Caution*: a warning against the registrant's name for up to five years.

- *Conditions of practice*: instructions that the registrant must follow to continue practising.

- *Suspension*: temporarily prevents the registrant practising for up to a year.

- *Strike from the register*: this can only be applied for misconduct or in the case of a conviction.

The panel may choose to take no further action – this is particularly likely where a registrant has engaged with the process, and has demonstrated remorse and remediation (in other words, has taken steps to ensure that the concern is unlikely to be repeated).

Self-referral

Before making a self-referral, it is important to cover the following points.

1. *Consider the need*: look at the HCPC (2024) *Standards of Conduct, Performance and Ethics* – section 9.5 highlights three key reasons to refer, specifically relating to criminal activity, regulator activity or employer restriction, suspension or dismissal. You should also refer if your health is impacting your ability to practise safely (section 6.3).

2. *Share the decision*: seek support from a trusted colleague or friend. Employer professional standards departments may be able to offer guidance, and consider organisations which may

provide legal support (such as the College of Paramedics or trade unions).

3. *Refer online*: a self-referral can be completed on the HCPC website, which will guide you through the correct steps and signpost you towards further support.

✏️ ACTIVITY

Search the Health and Care Professions Tribunal Service (HCPTS) website for examples of paramedic fitness to practise cases. Compare cases where no impairment was found with those where a sanction was applied, and reflect on the similarities and differences of each case.

Well-being and Resilience

Working as an NQP can be a highly rewarding experience, often viewed as a 'calling', and for this reason you may have made personal sacrifices to achieve your ambition of working as a paramedic. Unfortunately, these pressures do not stop at the point of registration, and you can find yourself struggling within your first year post qualification due to a misplaced belief that things will change. Although in some respects this will be true (there is nothing quite like the first month's wages after full-time education!), there are also many challenges associated with working as an NQP. Remaining cognisant of this, and implementing effective strategies to cope from the outset, are essential not just to support career longevity but also to ensure that you thrive, rather than simply survive, in the workplace. This section explores some of the common challenges you may experience.

Shift Work

The double-edged sword of long shifts and working unsocial hours can have a significant impact on you and your family. This can be exacerbated immediately following qualification by an eagerness to undertake additional hours (either financially motivated or due to enthusiasm for the role), which further reduces the rest and recovery time available. Employers often provide safeguards to manage this risk – including workload management tools, restrictions on rota design, minimum rest periods and attendance management policies – but when demand is high there is often an actual or perceived pressure to overlook these.

Practical steps which could help include the following:

- Ensure a clear delineation between work time and personal time, particularly through maintaining hobbies and relationships outside work.

- Avoid the temptation to undertake overtime, particularly in the early stages of a new role where cognitive demand is highest.

- Make use of organisational support mechanisms, such as flexible working arrangements and rota options.

- Maintain a consistent sleep schedule between shifts.

- Eat small amounts often during nightshifts to avoid energy dips. Avoid sugary snacks and energy drinks which provide a short-term boost, followed by a dip.

Coping Culture

Historically, there has been an expectation that paramedics 'just get on with it', and it has been culturally discouraged to raise concerns or highlight personal struggles, sometimes propagated through behaviour role-modelled by experienced employees who had moved into managerial roles. Despite a positive shift in attitudes, there are still many individuals who feel pressured to cope in the belief that this is in the best interests of their patients or colleagues.

Aside from the personal risks, this approach conversely increases the risk to patients, and many workplaces are now adopting initiatives which prioritise staff breaks over pure productivity. The HALT campaign pioneered by Guy's and St Thomas' (Baverstock and Finlay, 2019) recognises that where clinicians are **H**ungry, **A**ngry, **L**ate or **T**ired they are less productive and make poorer decisions, and encourages prioritising well-being by *halt*ing and taking breaks.

Intermittent Activity Intensity

The work you will undertake often involves episodes of very high physical, psychological and emotional demand, followed by periods of reduced activity (including low-acuity clinical work and organisational factors such as queuing to hand over or driving routinely into hospital). These peaks and troughs, coupled with the difficulty in predicting when the high-intensity moments will arise, can affect the way in which you process experiences and lead to increased stress and anxiety.

Emotional Trauma and Moral Injury

The average person will experience one or two deeply traumatic events during their lifetime, but for NQPs this figure is likely to be much higher, and so is the risk of consequential harm. Most paramedics have reported feeling deeply disturbed following a call and the prevalence rate of posttraumatic stress disorder (PTSD) is over 1 in 10, rising to 1 in 4 for general psychological distress (Petrie et al., 2018). For NQPs who are invariably experiencing a range of distressing events for the first time, often alongside junior colleagues who have equally little experience of emotional trauma, the impact can be significant.

Aside from PTSD, there is also significant risk of moral injury, where you experience a violation of your own code of ethics. This can occur through witnessing an event affecting another person (a form of vicarious trauma) or feeling forced to make a decision where there is no clear 'good' outcome, leading to feelings you 'should have done more'. Inexperience can lead to increased feelings of unjustified guilt, and recognising that this is unwarranted, as well as sharing your feelings with others, is essential to remediate the impact (Murray, 2019).

Following a traumatic event, symptoms such as flashbacks, intrusive thoughts, irritability, hypervigilance or numbness are common, but these will generally start to subside over a few weeks. It is important to be able to differentiate when these symptoms become prolonged or are having an adverse impact on either yourself or a colleague, to ensure appropriate professional help is sought.

Burnout and Compassion Fatigue

These two closely related but separate concerns are common not just within healthcare but across the wider workforce, with over three-quarters of workers in the UK reporting symptoms of burnout (Wickens, 2021). The World Health Organization (2019) recognises burnout as an occupational syndrome resulting from inadequately managed workplace stress, characterised by three elements:

- Exhaustion
- A negative or cynical outlook, often involving mental distancing
- Reduced professional efficacy.

Compassion fatigue occurs when burnout is combined with the physical and psychological impact of helping others, and can negatively impact both the professional and personal lives of those who experience it.

Since burnout is a cumulative phenomenon, it is less common for NQPs to experience it towards the start of their careers, but every individual has a different tolerance threshold for stress and the demands of emergency medicine can place you at a higher risk. The early symptoms of burnout can be similar to depression, and are often insidious and difficult to identify, highlighting the importance of remaining alert to symptoms in colleagues as much as in yourself.

Simple Techniques to Manage Well-being

Maintaining personal well-being is a complex but essential task, and there are a range of support services available to assist with this. Employers will generally provide occupational health and employee assistance programmes. Support is available through the NHS via a GP in the first instance, and there are various charities which offer specialist assistance to healthcare workers. The most important step for all these services is the first step – recognising the need and reaching out for help.

There are also some simple steps which can work as both preventive and restorative measures to improve well-being, and the following examples are offered as practical ways to prioritise your well-being.

- *Make a plan*: lifestyle changes are effective but can be difficult to implement and adhere to without a clear plan. Arrange activities with friends, be deliberate with downtime activities and protect time for hobbies.

- *Eat healthily*: fitting in healthy eating around a hectic work schedule can be challenging, but online resources to support healthy food choices and meal planning can help. Undertake healthy swaps, such as fruit or vegetables as snacks instead of sweets and chocolate.

- *Annual leave*: leave is an entitlement not a benefit but it is amazing how much annual leave is lost due to not being taken! Avoid undertaking overtime during annual leave if possible – a longer break from work to rest and recuperate offers significant benefits.

- *Say no*: NQPs are generally 'fixers' and naturally want to do all they can to help others, but it is important that this is not at the expense of your own well-being.

- *Sleep well*: small changes (such as presleep routines, keeping phones out of the bedroom and avoiding daytime naps) can have a positive impact on overall sleep quality.

- *Wake up early*: constantly hitting snooze and then rushing to get ready may feel like a good way to get more sleep, but it also increases stress and blood pressure. For early shifts, consider preparing the night before so that your morning is more serene.

- *Practise mindfulness*: this involves focusing on and accepting the present moment, without dwelling on what has happened in the past and what might happen in the future. It is commonly practised by taking time to pause and appreciate the simplicity of the here and now.

- *Acknowledge feelings*: it is normal for feelings to vary, and some days will inevitably be better than others – remember it's ok not to be ok. Sometimes just accepting this individually can be helpful, but if not then reach out to share your feelings with a trusted colleague or friend, or a support organisation such as the Samaritans.

- *Cut yourself some slack!* Despite the simplicity of some of these tips, they are not always easy to apply. Plans have a habit of changing, and even the healthiest person craves sugar from time to time. Remember, if something's worth doing, it's worth doing badly. While this sounds counterintuitive in a profession where continuous improvement is encouraged, it is important to have realistic expectations and celebrate small achievements. So, if you aimed to go on a 30-minute walk and only managed 15 minutes, remember that's better than no walk. If you aimed to replace all your snacks with fruit, but still ate a chocolate bar, commend yourself for eating more healthily than usual.

Chapter 8
Practice Education

In order to complete an accredited paramedic programme and join the paramedic register, you will have received a broad and varied educational input from many different sources. Some, such as university lecturers or trust education leads, will have been specifically recruited to assist with your learning journey. Others will have had no formal role in education, but will have shared the benefit of their experiences and been a positive role model for you. Often the most profound influence comes from practice educators (PEds, often referred to as mentors), and you can probably recall both positive and unsupportive experiences of the PEds you have worked with. Encouragingly, the constructive PEds tend to have the more lasting impact, and many experienced paramedics can still recall their most effective mentors during their training.

As you progress, the prospect of being responsible for, rather than receiving, practice education can seem daunting, particularly as preceptorship itself is a postregistration period of development. Despite this, it is important to acquire the awareness, skills and aptitude for practice education while an NQP to be fully prepared for working as an experienced paramedic.

Expectation

Historically, being a PEd was optional, and paramedics either volunteered or were nominated by their managers. The successful expansion of paramedic programmes, coupled with a drive by various organisations to improve the educational experience of students, has resulted in most employers expecting experienced paramedics to assume this role, and in 2016 the NHS introduced mentoring to the national job profile for experienced paramedics (NHS Staff Council, 2023). This is reflected in the HCPC (2023b) *Standards of Proficiency for Paramedics* which require paramedics to 'promote and engage in the learning of others' – an enhancement over the previous version which solely required an understanding of the importance of participation.

While the risks and benefits of enforcing the PEd role on reluctant participants are hotly debated, it remains clear that as the profession evolves, practice education will be an increasingly important, and required, component of paramedic practice. It is therefore sensible to focus on this during your supported developmental period.

> ### ADVICE
>
> 'I've found that being a PEd is an ideal way to maintain my own CPD – helping somebody learn is a huge motivation to learn more myself!'

Key Concepts in Supporting Learners in Practice

The paramedic profession is largely viewed as practical in nature, and with the increasingly academic focus on pre-registration education, the opportunity to apply theory to clinical practice cannot be overestimated. The role of the PEd is to guide the student through this integration, and the approach taken has a profound impact on learner success.

> ### ACTIVITY
>
> Consider which concepts from theory you found most difficult to apply in practice. What helped you to overcome the theory–practice divide?

There are various ways in which you can contribute to this as an NQP, and although the exact approach (and terminology used) will depend on your employer and working environment, the following concepts are noteworthy.

Supervision

Distinct from clinical supervision, in the PEd environment supervision refers to the direct observation of a learner applying a skill (both technical and non-technical) in practice. A primary principle of practice education is that the student learns from the experience of applying skills and knowledge they have been taught, and to do so requires the supervision of a suitably qualified clinician (since a student generally has no scope of practice to act independently). As a registered practitioner, an NQP can supervise a learner at any stage, and can usually sign to witness that a skill has been applied correctly (as well as confirming hours completed by a student, where this is required).

Supervision in practice does not imply any requirement to teach or guide, and you retain the right to withhold the opportunity for a student to perform an intervention which you do not feel confident supervising or would rather undertake yourself to benefit your own development. Factors affecting this decision will include the frequency with which the intervention is required, your experience, the potential risks associated and the ease of dynamically halting or reversing the actions of the student if necessary.

Guidance

Guidance or coaching is the next stage after supervision, whereby a student is offered advice on how to manage either the current or a future situation based on their performance. This could range from providing advice for subsequent encounters to talking through the stages of an intervention.

Coaching generally focuses on a specific aspect of development, as opposed to the overall performance of a student. Although there is no single correct method, it is considered more effective for a student to be guided towards reaching their own insight rather than being directed to the correct response (Starr, 2016). This aligns with the overarching intent of practice education which is to produce a well-rounded clinician, rather than a replica of the PEd.

Various models exist to support coaching conversations. Whitmore's (1992) GROW model is one of the most well known, but critics argue that it can be too transactional and that alternatives such as the FUEL model (Zenger and Stinnett, 2010) are more conversational and allow for greater flexibility (Table 8.1).

Table 8.1 – Two possible coaching models to support conversations.

GROW model (Whitmore, 1992)	FUEL model (Zenger and Stinnett, 2010)
Goal	**F**rame the conversation
Reality	**U**nderstand the current state
Options	**E**xplore the desired state
Will [do]	**L**ay out a success plan

Formative Assessment

A key distinction between supporting a learner and the role of the PEd is that of assessment – in other words, making a judgement regarding the individual's current, or future, performance against predetermined criteria. Although your role as an NQP in formative assessment depends on your organisation, it will usually only be expected once you have gained a degree of experience and confidence in your own practice, as well as training in the specifics of practice education and assessment. As a minimum, you should expect to have been shown the expectations of the learner's awarding organisation, including the assessment strategy and standard required, which are often stipulated within a practice assessment document (PAD). These vary considerably between universities and therefore being recently qualified may offer little reassurance of familiarity, and despite ongoing work by the College of Paramedics (2022b) to create a national PAD, this has not yet been widely adopted.

Formative assessment refers to the ongoing evaluation of a learner throughout a period of time (for example, a placement block), which is used to provide feedback and direct learning rather than contributing to a final result. Although the origins of the term are debated, this can be described as assessment *for* learning rather than assessment *of* learning – in other words, the emphasis is on identifying learning needs and opportunities rather than measuring the efficacy of that learning (Wiliam, 2011).

Undertaking formative assessment allows an introduction to the duties of the PEd, without the pressure of being responsible for the progression of a learner. This is particularly pertinent when the learner is underperforming, as it can be challenging for an NQP to inhibit progress of others while still focusing on their own development, leading to the risk of 'failure to fail' (Duffy, 2003).

Summative Assessment

Also referred to as 'end point assessment' (EPA) or 'sign off mentoring', the summative assessment is the summary judgement, usually at the end of a subject, module, placement block or course, where the PEd determines the student's ability to meet the relevant learning outcomes and fitness to practise against the HCPC standards. This is a significant responsibility, involving a degree of vicarious responsibility for the future actions and decisions of that student. For this reason, summative assessment rarely falls within the scope of practice of the NQP, although there is plenty of opportunity for you to support the decisions made by other PEds, which can be an effective way to gain the skills within a protected environment.

It is essential that PEds remain mindful of the professional implications of passing a learner who has not demonstrated the required standards, both for that individual and for the future patients they will treat. This leads many PEds to adopt an unofficial 'them and me' test.

- Would I want to work with this person?
- Would I want this person to treat my family?

While this can be a helpful guide to decision making and minimise the previously discussed danger of 'failure to fail', it can result in a higher 'pass' threshold being applied than is actually required. Ensuring the balance between meeting a minimum level of competence and recognising that all clinicians are fallible can be challenging, and needs to be applied objectively.

Even for experienced PEds, there is a concern that making judgements about the practice of others, as required by summative assessment, may lead to their own practice being scrutinised. A lack of confidence therefore leads to learners being given leeway even where they have not met the required standard (Sibson and Mursell, 2010). As an NQP this risk is greater, and therefore it is crucial that you seek, and receive, support prior to having summative mentoring included within your scope of practice.

Neurodiversity

First used in the 1990s, the term 'neurodiversity' describes the inherently varied ways in which individuals process the world around them. However, it is often used colloquially as an umbrella term to refer to neurodivergent individuals – those with neurodevelopmental conditions affecting cognition (Johnson and Ahluwalia, 2025). Prevalence amongst paramedics is not fully known, but several studies have established higher rates of specific conditions including attention deficit hyperactivity disorder (ADHD) and dyslexia within the emergency services (Davis, 2024; Lavender, 2017), which could imply a benefit to the unique strengths of neurodivergent individuals within such working environments.

> 💬 **ADVICE**
>
> 'As a PEd, I am always grateful when students share any neurodivergence – as well as demonstrating their trust in me, it allows me to continue developing inclusive teaching techniques which benefit everybody.'

Students and qualified paramedics who are neurodivergent may or may not have a formal diagnosis, and may or may not choose to share this information with others, often being concerned about the potential for discrimination. Regardless, adopting a strengths-based approach aligns with the social disability model which recognises that variations from the societal norm only disable an individual if the environment fails to match their needs. This places a moral imperative on clinicians and educators to provide an inclusive workplace which eventuates psychological safety for all. Support within the workplace is often available through occupational health and employee assistance programmes, and employers are legally obligated to provide reasonable adjustments to support employees who are neurodivergent.

✏️ ACTIVITY

Consider which of your character traits are most similar, and most different, to those of your colleagues. How do these differences enhance your practice as a clinician? How could you support colleagues who disclose they are neurodiverse?

💬 ADVICE

'Being diagnosed with dyslexia during my paramedic course came as a relief rather than a shock – I was able to understand why I'd struggled with some aspects of education previously and access the right support.'

Developing as a Practice Educator

Like many skills, the best way to develop as a PEd is to practise! Ideally, this would take place under the guidance of an experienced PEd who would be able to act as your 'practice educator' educator, but logistical and staffing restrictions often render this impractical. There are a range of opportunities for developing both mentoring and teaching skills and although not all will be available in every workplace, most areas will be open to a degree of collaboration between organisations.

Observing Mentoring in Practice

Although you will have experience of being the subject of mentoring, it can be helpful to watch other PEds undertake this role as an impartial observer (it is far easier to be objective about decisions when not directly affected by those decisions!). This can also be a valuable opportunity to discuss with experienced PEds how they developed their skills, and build on the experience of others. In particular, this can help with understanding how others make objective assessment decisions and communicate these to learners.

Undertake PEd Training

The availability and design of courses available vary by organisation, but best practice is to ensure NQPs are given training prior to becoming PEds. In 2023 the College of Paramedics launched an online course (available via e-Learning for Healthcare) which is designed to provide a consistent approach to PEd education. It is particularly helpful for NQPs as it provides a range of activities which can be undertaken to develop skills in practice.

Mentor Under Supervision

This can align with clinical supervision and allow you to develop your coaching skills with support. Even if this cannot be facilitated within your usual role, there may be opportunities to link in with trusts' education departments or local universities, who invariably seek support particularly with labour-intensive skills and simulation sessions.

Community Engagement

Schemes such as the Resuscitation Council 'Restart a Heart' campaign, local public access defibrillator initiatives and schools frequently seek support with delivering Basic Life Support (BLS) familiarisation, and this can offer an ideal opportunity for you to practise teaching in a supportive and positive environment.

Consider a situation where you have received feedback from someone you have been mentoring (either formally or informally). How has this changed your approach?

Inspiring Future Generations

The motivation to deliver practice education can be variable. Research undertaken when the PEd role was still voluntary suggested that there was an even split between those who undertook the role following a positive student experience and a subsequent desire to 'do their part' to pass this on, and those who had experienced such a poor approach that they sought to ensure future students did not suffer the same challenges (Clarke, 2018). The current integration of practice education within the paramedic role means this distinction is largely academic, and although there is some debate around the benefit realisation of reluctant mentors, this position is unlikely to change in the near future.

In reality, you will have amassed a range of experiences of practice education while a student, and will also have had circumstances which you initially perceived as unhelpful but have later recognised as significant to your development. While this should not in any way be seen as a defence of inappropriate PEd behaviour (which must never be tolerated), it does highlight that sometimes the recipient in the mentoring dyad needs to 'learn to learn' as much as the PEd needs to learn to mentor.

Having reached the milestone of qualifying as a paramedic, you may have begun seeking your next goal and often supporting students is a logical step. NQPs are sufficiently close to the student experience to be strong allies but are adequately experienced to be able to offer a qualified perspective (particularly due to the added accountability of professional registration). This can be a mixed blessing – inexperienced mentors are often outcome focused which can lead to the learner performing well but having insufficient understanding of what led to the outcome (Garvey, 2016). This, coupled with clinical inexperience, can mean the learner struggles to replicate a good outcome in future similar, but different, situations.

What is without question is that regardless of any formal expectation to support, coach or mentor students, you will inevitably be viewed as a role model by current students who will see you as the aspirational next step in their development – the goal the student is working towards. With this admiration comes a great deal of responsibility, and it is therefore incumbent on you to be a positive role model not just for student paramedics but for all those who you work alongside. Focusing on building others up can be a powerful tool in a profession which is often perversely focused on what has gone wrong, and receiving positive feedback can have a wide-reaching impact on both clinical performance and emotional well-being. It is in the ability to empower others that the true value of experience and mentorship lies. As an NQP, Barry Costello (2021) wrote of the 'outstanding' experienced clinicians he worked alongside: 'For all their knowledge, experience and advanced interventions, the skill I admired most was their ability to turn up to a challenging scene and empower an entire team of clinicians without even laying hands on the patient. As NQPs, there is no reason we shouldn't aim to emulate such leadership qualities in our everyday practice and work to build up those around us'. To do so does not require qualifications or experience, it simply requires compassion, grace and kindness – core values which can be demonstrated by all.

Epilogue

One of the privileges of my role within the ambulance service is the opportunity to attend the final day of induction courses for NQPs joining the Trust. This is always a celebration recognising the successes of those who are embarking on the next stages of their career, the difficulties that they may have had to overcome to reach this point, and the challenges which they might face moving forwards. The atmosphere is generally one of excitement, tinged with the mild terror which comes with facing the unknown. As I remind the graduating staff, many of the best clinicians I know will retain that excitement coupled with mild terror throughout their entire careers: the excitement keeps them enthusiastic and compassionate, and the terror keeps them safe.

I leave each cohort with two pieces of advice, both of which are pertinent to anybody moving into a new role regardless of where that may be, and therefore I consider them to be a fitting way to close this handbook. The first is to never be afraid to ask for help. Graduating as a paramedic marks the successful completion of a significant period of study and it is easy to assume that this means you are fully primed for every clinical and professional situation you may face. While this may be true, every clinician will face circumstances which they are unsure about or which cause them to doubt themselves, while new graduates often have a self-imposed expectation of knowledge which can be difficult to live up to. This is all the more significant if you are returning to work as a graduate paramedic where you have previously practised as a student. Be kind to yourself and ask the 'stupid' question – most of them turn out to be not so stupid after all. And by extension, never refuse help to someone who asks it of you – nobody knows the courage it takes to ask somebody a question they think they should know the answer to like an NQP!

Epilogue

The second piece of advice is to never forget the way you feel at the point of graduation. Being a paramedic can be an emotional rollercoaster – you can be subjected to the best and worst that humanity has to offer and can literally move from new life to end of life within an hour. Different working environments pose different challenges. It can be hard to retain your newfound enthusiasm when you're standing in the pouring rain at 4 o'clock in the morning during what feels like an endless run of nightshifts, but if you can maintain your passion and compassion in spite of these things, paramedicine is one of the best jobs in the world.

References

Bandali, M. (2022). Imposter syndrome. *Journal of Paramedic Practice*, 14(4), 172.

Bartlett, C. (2008). A tearoom view of mended ceramics. In: *Flickwerk: The Aesthetics of Mended Japanese Ceramics*. New York: Herbert F. Johnson Museum of Art, Cornell University and Münster: Museum für Lackkunst, pp. 18–24.

Bassford, C., Griffiths, F., Svantesson, M. *et al.* (2019). Developing an intervention around referral and admissions to intensive care: a mixed-methods study. *Health Service Delivery Research*, 7(39).

Baverstock, A. and Finlay, F. (2019). Take a break: HALT—are you Hungry, Angry, Late or Tired? *Archives of Disease in Childhood. Education and Practice Edition*, 104(4), 200.

Benner, P. (1984). *From Novice to Expert: Excellence And Power in Clinical Nursing Practice*. Menlo Park: Addison-Wesley.

Besco, R.O. (1995). To intervene or not to intervene? The Copilots "catch 22." Developing flight crew survival skills through the use of "P. A. C. E." In: Proceedings of the 25th International Seminar of the International Society of Air Safety Investigators Forum, 27(5), 94–101.

Best, M. and Neuhauser, D. (2004). Ignaz Semmelweis and the birth of infection control. *BMJ Quality and Safety*, 13, 233–234.

Birden, H., Glass, N., Wilson, I. *et al.* (2014). Defining professionalism in medical education: a systematic review. *Medical Teacher*, 36, 47–61.

Bravata, D.M., Watts, S A., Keefer, A.L. *et al.* (2020). Prevalence, predictors, and treatment of impostor syndrome: a systematic review. *Journal of General Internal Medicine*, 35, 1252–1275.

Burns, J.M. (1978). *Leadership*. New York: Harper and Row.

Clance, P.R. and Imes, S.A. (1978). The imposter phenomenon in high achieving women: dynamics and therapeutic intervention. *Psychotherapy*, 15(3), 241–247.

Clarke, V. (2018). The theory–practice relationship in paramedic undergraduate education. Unpublished doctoral thesis, University of Hertfordshire.

Clegg, D. and Barker, R. (1994). *Case Method Fast-Track: A RAD Approach*. Menlo Park: Addison-Wesley.

References

Clinical Human Factors Group (2005). *Just a routine operation*. Available at: https://chfg.org/chfg-history/

College of Paramedics (2021). *The Journey of the College of Paramedics*. Available at: https://collegeofparamedics.co.uk/COP/About_Us/The_Journey_of_the_College.aspx

College of Paramedics (2022a). *W.R.A.P.T.* Available at: https://wrap.collegeofparamedics.co.uk/

College of Paramedics (2022b). *College Knowledge*. Available at: https://collegeofparamedics.co.uk/COP/News/College_Knowledge/COP/News/College_Knowledge.aspx

College of Paramedics (2024a). *Paramedic Curriculum, 6th edn*. Available at: https://collegeofparamedics.co.uk/

College of Paramedics (2024b). *Paramedic Career Framework*. 5th edn revised. Bridgwater: College of Paramedics.

Cook, M.J. and Leathard, H.L. (2004). Learning for clinical leadership. *Journal of Nursing Management*, 12(6), 436–444.

Cooper, G.E., White, M.D. and Lauber, J.K. (1979). *Resource Management on the Flight Deck*. Moffett Field: NASA.

Costello, B. (2021). 'Fitting in' as an NQP. *Journal of Paramedic Practice*, 13(5), 216.

CQC (2015). *Defining 'Good' in Healthcare. Summary Report of Findings: Ambulance Services*. London: CQC.

CQC (2022). *Regulation 20: Duty of Candour*. London: CQC.

CQC (2024). *Single Assessment Framework*. London: CQC.

Dalai Lama (2021). *His Holiness the Dalai Lama's message to COP26*. Available at: https://www.dalailama.com/news/2021/his-holiness-the-dalai-lamas-message-to-cop26

Davis, D. (2024). Workforce diversity. *Journal of Paramedic Practice*, 16(10), 401.

Denning, S. (2014). *The Best of Peter Drucker*. New Jersey: Forbes.

Department of Health (2008). *A High-Quality Workforce: NHS Next Stage Review*. London: Department of Health.

Desveaux, L. and Ivers, N. (2024). Practice or perfect? Coaching for a growth mindset to improve the quality of healthcare. *BMJ Quality & Safety*, 33(4), 271–276.

Dewey, J. (1933). *How We Think: A Restatement of the Relation of Reflective Thinking to the Educative Process*. Boston: D.C. Heath & Co.

Dictionary.com (2025). *'Responsibility' and 'Accountable'*. Available at: dictionary.com

Donnelly, L. and Hamilton, L. (2012). A 'fresh eyes approach'. *Midwives*, 15(5), 44–45.

Downie, S., Walsh, J., Kirk-Brown, A. and Haines, T.P. (2023). How can scope of practice be described and conceptualised in medical and health professions? A systematic review for scoping and content analysis. *International Journal of Health Planning and Management*, 38(5), 1184–1211.

Drucker, P.F. (1992). *Managing for the Future*. Oxford: Routledge.

Duffy, K. (2003). *Failing Students: A Qualitative Study of Factors That Influence the Decisions Regarding Assessment of Students' Competence in Practice*. Glasgow: Caledonian Nursing and Midwifery Research Centre.

Dupont, G. (1997). The dirty dozen errors in maintenance. 11th Symposium on Human Factors in Aviation Maintenance.

Dweck, C.S. (2017). *Mindset: Changing the Way You Think to Fulfil Your Potential*. London: Robinson.

Eaton, G. (2023). Addressing the challenges facing the paramedic profession in the United Kingdom. *British Medical Bulletin*, 148, 70–78.

Equality Act 2010. Available at: www.legislation.gov.uk/ukpga/2010/15/contents

Express and Star (2023). Demise of private ambulance firm. Available at: www .expressandstar.com/news/local-hubs/staffordshire/cannock/2023/01/19/demise -of-private-ambulance-firm-with-cannock-headquarters-sees-150-jobs-lost/

First, S., Tomlins, L. and Swinburn, A. (2012). From trade to profession – the professionalisation of the paramedic workforce. *Journal of Paramedic Practice*, 4(7), 378–381.

Gale, C.P. (2017). Acute coronary syndrome in adults: scope of the problem in the UK. *British Journal of Cardiology*, 24(s1), 3–9.

Garvey, B. (2016). When mentoring goes wrong.... In: Clutterbuck, D. and Lane, G. (eds) *The Situational Mentor*. Farnham: Gower Press, pp. 160–177.

Gawunde, A. (2009). *The Checklist Manifesto*. New York: Metropolitan Books.

Goldsmith, M. (2002). Try feedforward instead of feedback. *Leader to Leader*, 25, 11–14.

Greenaway, R., Vaida, B. and Iepure, C. (2015). *Active Reviewing: A Practical Guide for Trainers and Facilitators*. Charleston: CreateSpace.

Greenhalgh, T. (2010). *How to Read a Paper: The Basics of Evidence-Based Medicine*. Hoboken: John Wiley and Sons.

Hampton, J.R. (1983). The end of clinical freedom. *BMJ*, 287, 1237–1238.

Handyside, B. and Watson, K. (2023). The experiences of and attitudes towards continuing professional development: an interpretative phenomenological analysis of UK paramedics. *Emergency Medicine Journal*, 40(s1), A7.

Hayes, T. (2022). *Why UK Paramedics are Leaving Ambulance Services to Work Clinically Elsewhere in the NHS*. Nuneaton: Association of Ambulance Chief Executives Ambulance Leadership Forum.

References

HCPC (2014). *Professional Indemnity and Your Registration.* London: HCPC.

HCPC (2017). *Continuing Professional Development and Your Registration.* London: HCPC.

HCPC (2021). *HCPC Diversity Data Report 2021: Paramedics.* Available at: www .hcpc-uk.org/globalassets/resources/factsheets/hcpc-diversity-data-2021 -factsheet--paramedics.pdf

HCPC (2023a). *Principles for Preceptorship.* London: HCPC.

HCPC (2023b). *Standards of Proficiency for Paramedics.* London: HCPC.

HCPC (2024). *Standards of Conduct, Performance and Ethics.* London: HCPC.

HCPC (2025). *Registrant Snapshot.* Available at: www.hcpc-uk.org/resources/ data/2025/registrant-snapshot-april-2025/

HCPC and College of Paramedics (2020). *A joint statement of support for paramedics.* Available at: www.hcpc-uk.org/registrants/updates/2020/a-joint-statement -of-support-for-paramedics/

Health Education England (2018). *RePAIR: Reducing Pre-Registration Attrition and Improving Retention Report.* London: HEE.

Health Education England (2021). *Results Overview Advanced Practice, The HEE National Education and Training Survey (NETS).* Available at: https://advanced -practice.hee.nhs.uk/wp-content/uploads/sites/28/2022/04/AP-NETS-Results -Report-Nov-2021.pdf

Henderson, T., Endacott, R., Marsden, J. and Black, S. (2019). Examining the type and frequency of incidents attended by UK paramedics. *Journal of Paramedic Practice*, 11(9), 396–402.

Hersey, P. and Blanchard, K.H. (1969). Life cycle theory of leadership. *Training & Development Journal*, 23(5), 26–34.

Howlett, G. (2019). Nearly qualified student paramedics' perceptions of reflection and use in practice. *Journal of Paramedic Practice*, 11(6), 258–263.

Institute of Medicine (2000). *To Err is Human: Building a Safer Health System.* Washington, DC: National Academies Press.

Johnson, J. and Ahluwalia, S. (2025). Neurodiversity in the healthcare profession. *Postgraduate Medical Journal*, 101(1192), 167–171.

Joint Emergency Services Interoperability Principles (JESIP) (2024). *Joint Doctrine: The Interoperability Framework 3.1.* Available at: www.jesip.org.uk/downloads/ joint-doctrine-guide/

Kent Online (2024). *Staff in shock as Dartford-based private ambulance company ceases trading.* Available at: www.kentonline.co.uk/dartford/news/ we-are-all-in-shock-staff-furious-as-ambulance-firm-cease-312124/

Kirkebøen, G. (2009). Decision behaviour-improving expert judgement. In: Williams, T.M., Samset, K. and Sunnevåg, K.J. (eds) *Making Essential Choices with Scant Information*. Basingstoke: Palgrave Macmillan.

Klein, G.A. (1998). *Sources of Power: How People Make Decisions*. Cambridge: MIT Press.

Korczynski, M. (2003). Communities of coping: collective emotional labour in service work. *Organization*, 10(1), 55–79.

Kramer, M. (1975). Reality shock: why nurses leave nursing. *American Journal of Nursing*, 75(5), 891.

Lark (2023). *STAR method*. Available at: www.larksuite.com/en_us/topics/productivity-glossary/star-method

Lave, J. and Wenger, E. (1991). *Situated Learning: Legitimate Peripheral Participation*. Cambridge: Cambridge University Press.

Lavender, R.J. (2017). What can dyslexic paramedic students teach us about mentoring? A case study. *Journal of Paramedic Practice*, 9(5), 202–206.

Lawrence-Wilkes, L. and Ashmore, L., (2014). *The Reflective Practitioner in Professional Education*. Basingstoke: Palgrave Macmillan.

Lewin, K., Lippitt, R. and White, R.K. (1939). Patterns of aggressive behavior in experimentally created "social climates". *Journal of Social Psychology*, 10(2), 269–299.

Limmer, D. (2015). *Evolution of the confident EMS provider*. Available at: https://limmereducation.com/article/evolution-of-the-confident-ems-provider/

The Lion King (1994). [Film] Directed by R. Allers and R. Minkoff. USA: Walt Disney Pictures.

Lombardo, C., Dawe, J., Austin, E. *et al*. (2024). Staff and patient insights to improve fatigue management in NHS ambulance services: CATNAPS study. *British Paramedic Journal*, 9(2), 62–63.

Mallinson, T. (2020). Clinical courage. *Journal of Paramedic Practice*, 12(11), 429.

Mann, R.D. (1959). A review of the relationships between personality and performance in small groups. *Psychological Bulletin*, 56(4), 241–270.

McClelland, G., Burrow, E., Alton, A. *et al*. (2023). What factors contribute towards ambulance on-scene times for suspected stroke patients? An observational study. *European Stroke Journal*, 8(2), 492–500.

McNicoll, A. (2008). *Peer supervision – no-one knows as much as all of us*. Available at: https://www.coachingmentoring.co.nz/articles/peer-supervision-no-one-knows-much-all-us

Melia, S. (2024). *Culture Review of Ambulance Trusts*. London: NHS.

References

Murray, E. (2019). Moral injury and paramedic practice. *Journal of Paramedic Practice*, 11(10), 424–425.

National Patient Safety Agency (2003). *The Incident Decision Tree*. London: NPSA.

Newton, A. (2012). The ambulance service: the past, present and future. *Journal of Paramedic Practice*, 4(6), 365–368.

NHS (2023). *NHS Long Term Workforce Plan*. Available at: www.england.nhs.uk/publication/nhs-long-term-workforce-plan/

NHS Employers (2017). *Principles of the Newly Qualified Paramedic Consolidation of Learning Programme*. London: NHS Employers.

NHS England (2023a). *Allied Health Professions (AHP) Preceptorship Standards and Framework*. London: NHS.

NHS England (2023b). *Paramedic Leadership in Ambulance Trusts in England*. London: NHS.

NHS England (2024). *National Flexible Working People Policy Framework*. Available at: www.england.nhs.uk/long-read/national-flexible-working-people-policy-framework/

NHS Institute for Innovation and Improvement (2010). *Safer Care*. London: NHS.

NHS Staff Council (2016). *Implementation of the New Band 6 Paramedic Profile in Ambulance Trusts in England*. London: NHS.

NHS Staff Council (2023). *National Profiles for Ambulance Service*. London: NHS.

NICE (2018). *Principles for Putting Evidence-based Guidance into Practice*. London: NICE.

Osborne, S. (2015). The standard you walk past is the standard you accept. *ACORN*, 28(2), 26–27.

Petrie, K., Milligan-Saville, J., Gayed, A. *et al.* (2018). Prevalence of PTSD and common mental disorders amongst ambulance personnel: a systematic review and meta-analysis. *Social Psychiatry and Psychiatric Epidemiology*, 53, 897–909.

Phillips, P. (2024). Becoming a paramedic: the experiences of newly qualified paramedics in navigating a changing professional, social, and personal identity. PhD thesis, Bournemouth University.

Pollock, K. (2013). *Review of Persistent Lessons Identified Relating to Interoperability from Emergencies and Major Incidents since 1986*. Easingwold: Emergency Planning College.

Povich, S. (1997). *The ball stayed white, but the game did not*. Available at: https://www.washingtonpost.com/wpsrv/sports/longterm/general/povich/launch/jackier.htm

Race, P. (2001). *Using Feedback to Help Students to Learn.* Available at: https://phil-race.co.uk/wp-content/uploads/Using_feedback.pdf

Reason, J. (1997). *Managing the Risks of Organizational Accidents.* Farnham: Ashgate Publishing.

Ridings, J.E. (2013). The thalidomide disaster, lessons from the past. In Felix, L. (ed.) *Teratogenicity Testing: Methods and Protocols.* Champaign: Humana Press, pp. 575–586.

Rolfe, G., Freshwater, D. and Jasper, M. (2001). *Critical Reflection in Nursing and the Helping Professions: A User's Guide.* Basingstoke: Palgrave Macmillan.

Sampson, F.C., O'Hara, R., Long, J. and Coster, J.E. (2024). Understanding good communication in ambulance pre-alerts to Emergency Department. Findings from a qualitative study of UK emergency services. *BMJ Open*, 15, e094221.

Sibson, L. and Mursell, I. (2010). Mentorship for paramedic practice: bridging the gap. *Journal of Paramedic Practice*, 2(6), 270–274.

Snowdon, K. (2021). Exploring the clinical debrief: benefits and barriers. *Journal of Paramedic Practice*, 13(1), 1–7.

Starr, J. (2016). *The Coaching Manual.* Harlow: Pearson.

Titler, M.G. (2006). Developing an evidence-based practice. In LoBiondo-Wood, G. and Haber, J. (eds) *Nursing Research: Methods and Critical Appraisal for Evidence-based Practice*, 7th edn. St Louis: Mosby, pp. 385–437.

Tuttle, J.E. and Hubble, M.W. (2018). Paramedic out-of-hospital cardiac arrest case volume is a predictor of return of spontaneous circulation. *Western Journal of Emergency Medicine*, 19(4), 654–659.

van der Gaag, A., Gallagher, A., Zasada, M. *et al.* (2017). *People Like Us? Understanding Complaints about Paramedics And Social Workers.* Final Report, University of Surrey.

Vít, M., Kučera, J., Lenárt, P. *et al.* (2023). Biological factors and self-perception of stress in relation to freeze-like response in humans. *Psychoneuroendocrinology*, 158, 106382.

Vygotsky, L.S. (1978). *Mind in Society: The Development of Higher Psychological Processes.* Cambridge: Harvard University Press.

Whitmore, J. (1992). *Coaching for Performance: A Practical Guide to Growing Your Own Skills.* London: Nicholas Brealey Publishing.

Wickens, Z. (2021). *79% of UK staff have gone through burnout.* Available at: https://employeebenefits.co.uk/79-uk-staff-gone-through-burnout/

Wiliam, D. (2011). What is assessment for learning? *Studies in Educational Evaluation*, 37(1), 3–14.

References

Wise, J. (1991). *Career Comeback: Taking Charge of Your Career.* Melbourne: Pitman.

World Health Organization (2019). QD85 Burnout. In *International Statistical Classification of Diseases and Related Health Problems*, 11th edn. Geneva: WHO.

Wright, J. Jr. and Schachar, N.S. (2020). Necessity is the mother of invention: William Stewart Halsted's addiction and its influence on the development of residency training in North America. *Canadian Journal of Surgery*, 63(1), E13–19.

Zenger, J. and Stinnett, K. (2010). *The Extraordinary Coach: How the Best Leaders Help Others Grow.* London: McGraw-Hill Education.

Index

Index

www.ingramcontent.com/pod-product-compliance
Lightning Source LLC
Chambersburg PA
CBHW061255220326
41599CB00028B/5662